'A RARE HE

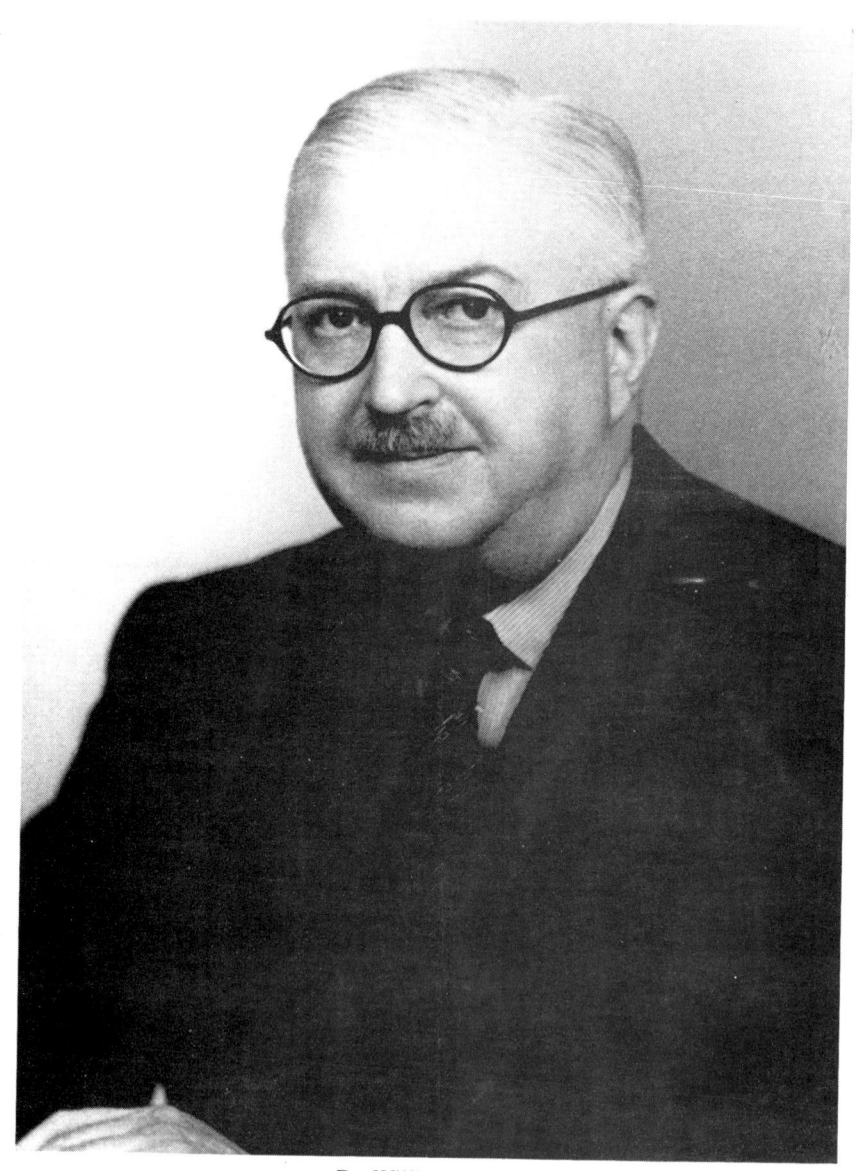

Dr. William Evans.

# 'A RARE HERO'
## Dr William Evans

D.Sc(Lond) M.D., F.R.C.P., Hon D.Sc(Wales)

24.11.1895 - 20.9.1988

BUDDUG OWEN

GEE & SON LIMITED
DENBIGH

*First Impression: October 1999*

ISBN 0 7074 0329 4

✧

Dedicated to

RICHARD and EIDDWEN PHILLIPS

my parents

whose encouragement and support

allowed me to open my own furrow.

✧

*Printed and Published by*
GEE & SON LIMITED, DENBIGH, N. WALES

# Contents

# Acknowledgements

The instigator of this book is Miss Frances Evans, Dr William Evans' niece, and I am indebted to her for giving of her time and energy, hospitality and access to Dr Evans' papers, manuscripts, articles and books. I have written to or spoken to many people about Dr Evans and they include, Roderic Bowen, Wallace Brigden, Brian Cooke, Sheila Cross, John Cule, Arthur Hollman, Les Hughes, Huw Edwards, Emyr Wyn Jones, Aubrey Leatham, Megan Lewis, Mair Owen, Bethan Phillips, W. J. St. E-G Rhys, Jane Roderic-Evans, Malcolm Towers, Donald Williams and Elizabeth Williams. All provided helpful information or pointed me in the right direction. Sian M. Drake – Assistant Librarian, Bibliographic Data Management Division and Cyril Evans – Cataloguing Assistant, Department of Manuscripts and records of the National Library of Wales were helpful with references as was Jonathan Evans, Archivist at the Royal London Hospital.

My husband, Elwyn Owen typed the manuscript. Emlyn Evans and Alun Williams of Gwasg Gee have been helpful and accommodating. To all, and others whom I have inadvertently left out I wish to express my gratitude. Dr Evans, as a countryman wrote about the Plough. I hope I have opened a furrow on his life and work which merits further more detailed research than I have given.

*Buddug Owen*
August 1999

Chapter 1

# Introduction

My title is taken from an obituary of Dr William Evans written by David Mendel[1] for the Independent Newspaper. When Dr Evans was 90 his friend and colleague Dr Byron Evans organised a birthday celebration for him in Cardiff and circularised his former assistants urging early application to the party. At that time Dr Evans had been retired for 25 years but admiration and affection brought almost all his surviving assistants to Cardiff in mid November. As Mendel wrote 'It is a rare hero who commands that sort of loyalty'.

When I consulted the Dictionary for the meaning of 'Hero' I found several definitions but the one I liked best to sum him up was 'a man who is idealised for possessing superior qualities in any field'. As the obituary said 'Integrity, humanity, intelligence and wit, all in unusually high dosage, had combined to make him the complete doctor; skilled, well loved by the patients, a hero to his assistants and students and an innovator'.

He was a kind, helpful, courteous, compassionate, loveable and dynamic man who did not talk a lot or show off, was easy to confide in but difficult to get to know. A 'Cardi' who had native Welsh shrewdness and intuition, was single minded and had iron self-discipline, did not court favours nor receive honours but could be devastating in judgement. A noted raconteur, he taught like a lay-preacher seeming to come alive in the Consulting Room and was full of witty one-liners.

Born in a farmhouse just outside Tregaron, his name appears on the Roll of Honour on a Board in the Memorial Hall as one of a number who served in the First World War. He became one of the foremost Cardiologists of his time in London who attended the National Heart Hospital and had an international influence on postgraduate students.

[1] Mendel, D. Obituary Dr William Evans – Independent Newspaper 24 Sept. 1988.

On retiring from active practice he returned to spend the last 21 years of his life in Tregaron tending his roots and becoming involved in all aspects of life in this place. I met him once when I accompanied my sister to Bryndomen and was shown his tool shed where everything was tidily and methodically displayed in its correct place. I was impressed and remember at the time thinking that he had a precise orderly mind.

Some two years ago I was asked whether I would be interested in writing his biography and felt diffident about this. It was not made easier when I was told by a former colleague of his that he was a superb writer who had written his Autobiography and really – was there a need for a Biography?

Also an article by Dr Ivor Felstein[2] on writing for medical publications gave Dr William Evans with Dr Richard Asher, as a superb example of a successful medical writer with characteristics of keeping sentences short, adjectives limited, sequences logical, does not digress from the agreed topic, clearly explains unusual terms and concepts, strictly limits all forms of jargon, adheres to the editorially agreed format and provides meticulous references during and at the end of articles.

When I met his niece Miss Frances Evans at her home in Tyndomen I became enthralled by her Uncle's life and times as well as by her own interests in the country, rural life, farming and the environment and by her determination to save the best of the past. Miss Evans has been generous in allowing me access to Dr Evans papers and I have regarded it as a privilege to visit Tyndomen and to get the feel of their life when he retired from London.

[2] Felstein, I. "The Gentle but difficult art of writing for medical publications'. Rostrum (Pfizer Ltd.) 1982. No. 106 p. 23-24.

Chapter 2

# Early Years

He was born on 24 November 1895 in Tyndomen, Tregaron, a farmhouse some mile and a half from the town of 700 population at the time.

His imagination had been captured as a child by his Maternal grandfather Joseph Jenkins whose diary he was to notate and publish years later as the 'Diary of a Welsh Swagman'.[3] Joseph was 80 and a frail broken man but to a child a romantic figure, a man who had farmed Trecefel, one of the best farms in Cardiganshire which was next to Tyndomen. A visionary and forceful leader who was interested in education and who was instrumental in building and equipping the first modern school in the district in 1857 for 450 children aged between 5-16 years. A poet known as Amnon 11, he formed an Adult Literary Society which held weekly Essay Competitions. He was a Diarist from the age of 21 in 1839 until 1894 – a span of 55 years. He campaigned successfully to persuade Manchester and Milford Railway Co. to lay a track to connect Carmarthen and Aberystwyth with a station at Tregaron. Yet, when he was 51 years old he emigrated to Australia for 25 years returning to spend the last three years of his life with his family in Trecefel where he died aged 80 in 1898.

Dr Evans indicates that it was a nagging wife who forced him to leave home but Bethan Phillips[4] in her interesting Biography of Joseph 'Rhwng Dau Fyd' lays the blame on alcohol for the deteriorating relationship with his family, especially his wife, for his sudden decision to leave. This book won 3rd prize in the Welsh Booker Prize at Hay-on-Wye Literary Festival in 1999.

Dr Evans came from farming stock on both sides though there were doctors in the family. Joseph Jenkins' youngest son John David qualified in 1897 while his wife Elizabeth's brother had 2 sons who

---

[3] Evans, W. 'Diary of a Welsh Swagman' – Sun Australia 1975.
[4] Phillips, B. 'Rhwng Dau Fyd' Cymdeithas Lyfrau Ceredigion 1998.

were doctors, Dr Evan Evans of Greengrove and Aeron Villa, a General Practitioner; and Dr Tom Evans, MOH Swansea. Elizabeth had been bequeathed a considerable inheritance and did not want to see this inheritance squandered by her husband's behaviour. His Mother Elinor 1853-1924 called Nel, Joseph and Elizabeth's 4th child was born at Trecefel and educated privately in Knighton. She was a self-reliant lady who could turn her hand to anything and supervised the building of the new farmhouse at Tyndomen, grew shrubs and flowers which were foreign to the district as well as being a good needle woman. She and her husband Ebenezer 1845-1922 had five children, three boys and two girls. Their eldest daughter Elizabeth called Lizzie (1880-1925) married and died at Nantgaredig; one son Ieuan died at Tyndomen aged seven from Scarlet Fever, the second daughter Margaret 1884-1888 died young and the remaining two sons Joseph 1893-1969 and William 1895-1988 grew to adulthood. (Family Tree – Fig. 1)

William chronicled his childhood in great detail in his Autobiography[5] and recognises the great debt he owed to his parents. Sundays were strictly observed and though his father was a Calvinistic Methodist and mother an Unitarian he and his brother were brought up in the Church of England (before disestablishment) for the probable reason that to get a bursary to proceed with higher education the child had to belong to the church. Grace was said before meals and Bible reading and prayers afterwards. Truthfulness and compassion were instilled into the children from an early age. He read a Chapter of the Bible before retiring throughout his life.

Before the move to secondary education he and his brother had to decide who was going to remain on the farm. His brother was the elder and could plough a straight furrow and opted for the land to William's disappointment as he was interested in the countryside. The one who opted for farming was to be given private education at Llandovery College, the other to go to the local County School. William had a bursary to go there in 1911 and though he was interested in Science it was planned that he should enter a Divinity College after Matriculation. He did well in Greek and secured a place in Lampeter College but disestablishment of the Church convinced his father that clergy stipend would be jeopardised and advised William not to take up the place. He had matriculated in 1913 in eight subjects including

[5] Evans, W. 'Journey to Harley Street' – David Rendel Ltd. London 1968.

Greek and Latin, won prizes in drawing and debating and had been practising giving sermons in the barn using a sack of corn as pulpit and so was disappointed. 50 years later he was to preach in Llandaff Cathedral and St. Martin's in the Fields in London as representative of the Chest and Heart Foundation.

He was invited when he was High Sheriff to speak at his school's Speech Day[6] and spoke of the standards which had been set for him as a child. He pointed out that Genius may never get you to the top but continuous plodding will. He asked the children to take ten vows with him which he called the commandments of Wayside Religion or Good Manners.

Manners are not trivial but a duty as a citizen and conventional courtesy. They have to be learnt and practised before they become second nature.

1. Close doors not slam them. Noise causes irritability but quietness will help one to walk through life graciously and with dignity.
2. To rise from your seat for a lady or your seniors when they walk into the room is a symbol of maturity.
3. Give up your seat for a lady or your elders in public transport.
4. Walk on the outside of a lady on the pavement and cultivate a samaritan spirit.
5. Cultivate good table manners.
6. Always be neat and tidy. (A Lady Doctor applied for a post and on leaving the interview it was noticed that the seam of her stocking was not straight. She did not get the job!).
7. Be punctual.
8. Acknowledge all letters promptly.
9. Write bread and butter letters.
10. Cultivate speaking to the lonely' etc. This brings joy to others and helps to smooth the path of life.

Assiduity is what pays in the end.

He also encouraged them to specialise in four things – an occupation, one of the Arts, a Hobby, and a Solitarium or Quiet Place to cultivate the soul.

He quoted the last words of Walter Scott to his son-in-law on his death bed 'Be a good man, nothing else will give you comfort when you come to lie here'.

[6] Evans, W. 'Wayside Religion' – National Farmers Union – Cardiganshire County Branch 1960 Year Book p. 47-57.

He and his brother improvised on the farm. They made a boat which sank and from which he was rescued as he could not swim and also made a static bicycle which he remembered later as a prototype for a scientific ergometer in the Physiology Laboratory to test the effect of physical exercise on respiratory and circulatory function.

Animals became friends and in a paper to the British Goat Society[7] he extolled the virtue of children caring for goats in order to have an efficient milk supply for a rural population. This paper was given to help an Uncle who had a rural practice and who was concerned about his patients' health. In 1934 he spoke in favour of clean milk without coliform contamination but thought a little Tubercle for a child was a help to withstand the disease and was not in favour of Tuberculin free milk. This was against contemporary thought.

He had two accidents with horses, in one suffering a crushed leg and broken collar bone and the other a crushed arm. He enjoyed hunting, fishing, playing football using an inflated pig's bladder and using a discarded perambulator as a go-cart.

Having been discouraged from entering the Church by his father, his Bank Manager tried to discourage him from entering the Bank because of the long hours, responsibilities and poor pay. He had to take an entrance exam because the Welsh Matriculation did not exempt him from this and he started as a junior clerk in the Dowlais Branch of Lloyds Bank in 1914 after going to London for a medical examination where he was told he had Scoliosis but was otherwise fit for work. His starting salary was £40 per annum and he had to dress immaculately, sporting a watch on a gold chain across his waistcoat. Here he says he learnt to be courteous, chatty with customers, have legible and tidy handwriting, be accurate with all ledger entries and all filing procedures. These attributes remained lifelong; perhaps he was obsessively tidy and methodical. In two years he had become 2nd cashier and as Deputy for the Manager he was issued with an Air-Gun! One of his first lessons was to be sure to stick stamps straight on envelopes.

He undertook a Correspondence Course to sit the Institute of Bankers examination but his studies were interrupted by the War and never resumed. 40 years later he was appointed the first Consulting Cardiologist to Messrs Lloyds Bank.

---

[7] Evans, W. A plea for a more efficient milk supply for our Rural Populace – British Goat Society.

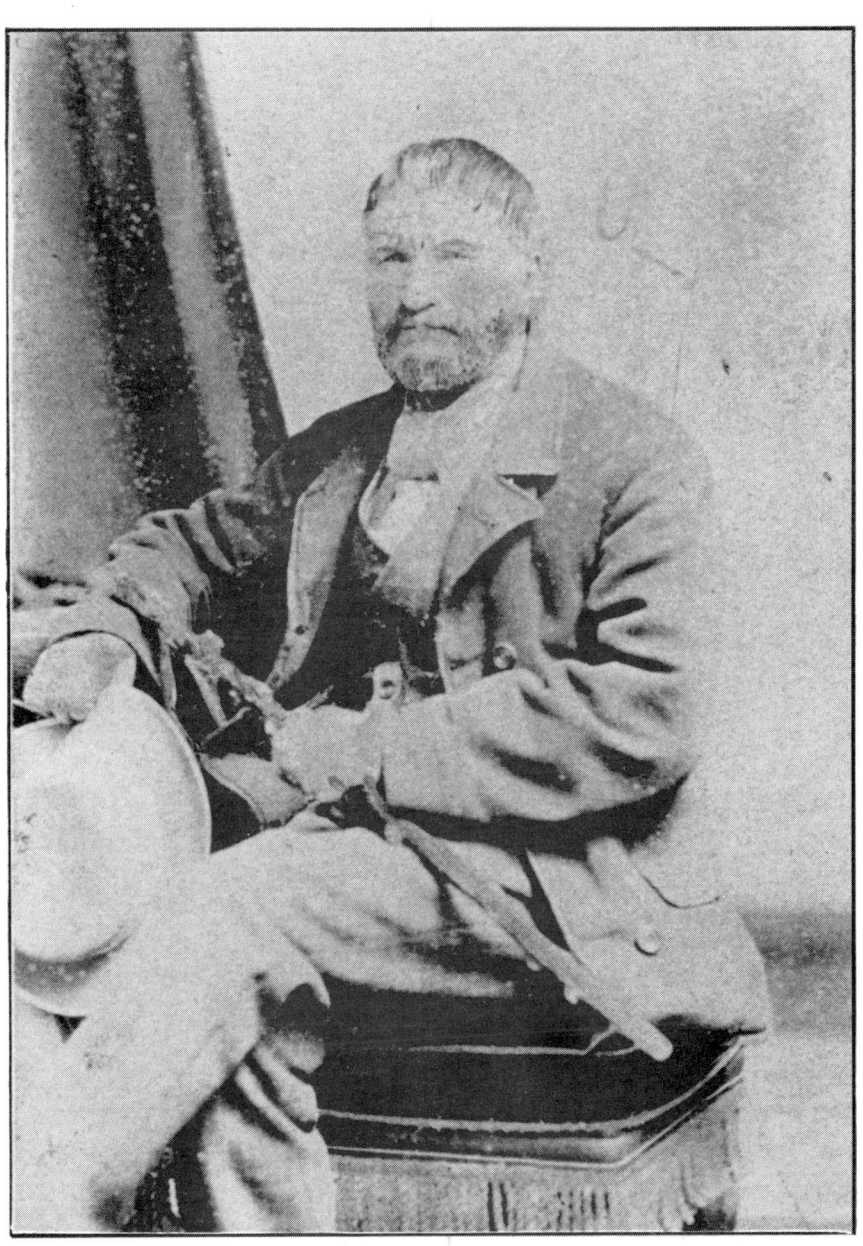

Joseph Jenkins, Trecefel.
*(Photograph by permission of Miss Frances Evans.)*

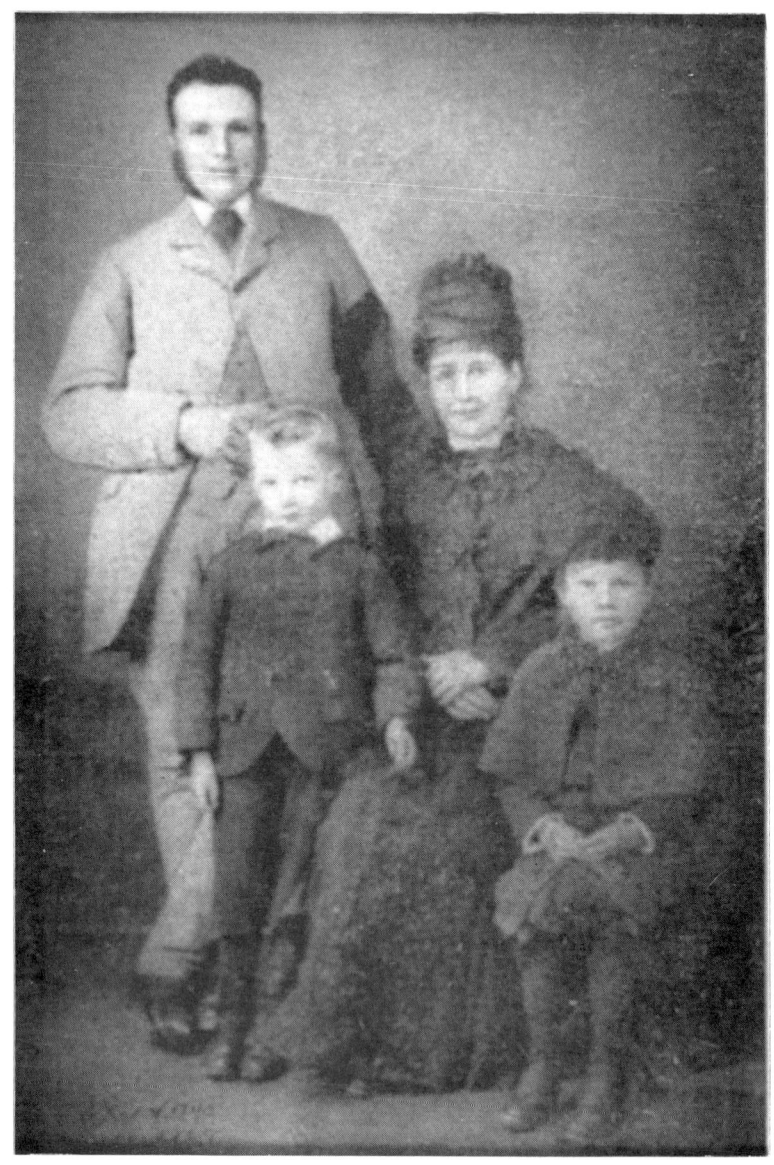

Ebenezer and Elinor Evans, Ieuan and Lizzie.
*(Photograph by permission of Miss Frances Evans.)*

He entered the Bankers Battalion, the Second-fifth Buffs on 28 April 1916, as a private and was selected for Commission entering the Cadet School at Peterhouse College, Cambridge and gazetted to the Lancashire Fusiliers, After a month's training as Infantry Officer he was sent to France, seeing action in Ypres and the Battle of Passchendaele. He embarked for France on 11 October 1917 his first sight being a two mile queue of Ambulances carrying wounded to the hospital ship and where he was affected the following morning by reading that three men were to be shot at dawn having been convicted of desertion by Courts Martial. This had a great affect on him and he took a personal interest in all men in his charge and got a man of his own platoon acquitted of the same charge from the knowledge he had of him and his problems through reading his Correspondence. Through this personal knowledge he was able to gain their loyalty, devotion and discipline. He lost four batmen in 18 months and was affected by the acts of heroism and chivalry he witnessed. He was missing for a time and also was gassed and had to be removed from the Front. He was partly electrocuted when a wiring party was struck by Lightning and four of his men killed. Once when he returned from leave he found only three of his platoon of thirty had survived and felt 'the flower of the Battalion had wilted'. During his time at the Front he wrote poetry which he sent home and although I read that he had published a volume of poetry Miss Evans tells me that this is not so although he did get some published in newspapers. He won a prize at a St. David's day Eisteddfod in 1918 for a poem. At the end of the war he was gazetted Battalion Education Officer to assist in demobilisation and resettlement and was demobilised on 21 August 1919.

He had decided to pursue a professional career in Medicine instead of Banking and on discharge his Confidential Report read 'A most capable officer of good professional knowledge. Recommended for promotion. A good instructor. A good leader. An excellent disciplinarian. Daring in action'.

He had experience of First Aid in the Army and although he was tempted to make the Army his career he felt that as he had not gained a decoration he would not be able to advance for promotion. His name though appears on the Roll of Honour in the Memorial Hall in Tregaron.

Chapter 3

# Medical Training

At the end of the war he was 23 years old and had saved £600, and decided to pursue a career in Medicine. He entered UCW Aberystwyth in October 1919, took the London Matriculation in January 1920 and in July the 1st M.B. in Botany, Zoology, Physics and Chemistry. Only 4 of 16 finished the course because of the difficulty they found in settling to study.

In September 1920 he applied for admission to the London Hospital and commenced his medical studies the following month without a selection interview. After eighteen months he started clinical work and got a stethoscope which 'gave one prestige and we sported it prominently round the neck'. Each student was allotted a share in the care of 6-12 patients and designated 'clerk to the case' or 'dresser' if the patient had a surgical problem. He had a high regard for his teachers. He qualified in the Autumn of 1924 with MRCS, LRCP and in May 1925 MB, BS with Honours in Surgery having enjoyed his student days and by careful living and Government Grant for Medical College fees he finished with £34 in the bank. He had gained the Outpatient Dressers Prize in 1921 and the Inpatient Dressers Prize in 1922.

He thought he was unworthy to work in the London and got an appointment in Queen Mary's Hospital, Stratford as Casualty Officer and House Physician commencing 1 July 1925. After six weeks he had a rectal haemorrhage and was admitted to hospital for six weeks. When he returned to his post he found it had been filled as it had been assumed he would never be fit enough to return.

He became a locum in General Practice in Surrey and applied for a post as Medical Officer of Health in Cardiganshire in late 1925[8] and also for a post of Assistant to the Professor of the Pathology Department London Hospital. He gained the Pathology post starting

---

[8] Evans, W. Personal Papers.

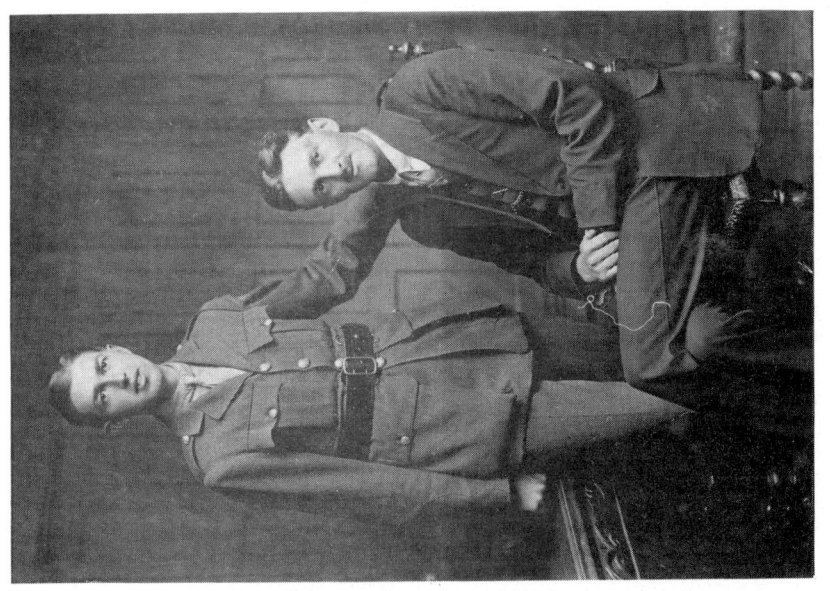

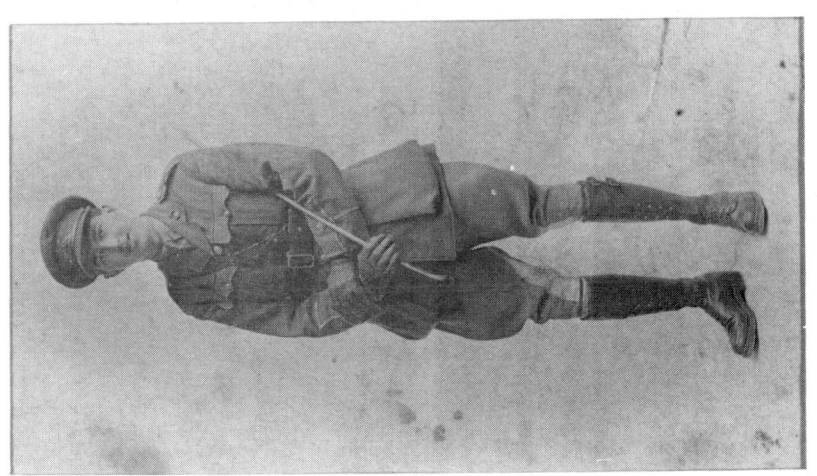

Army Days.

*(Photographs by permission of Miss Frances Evans.)*

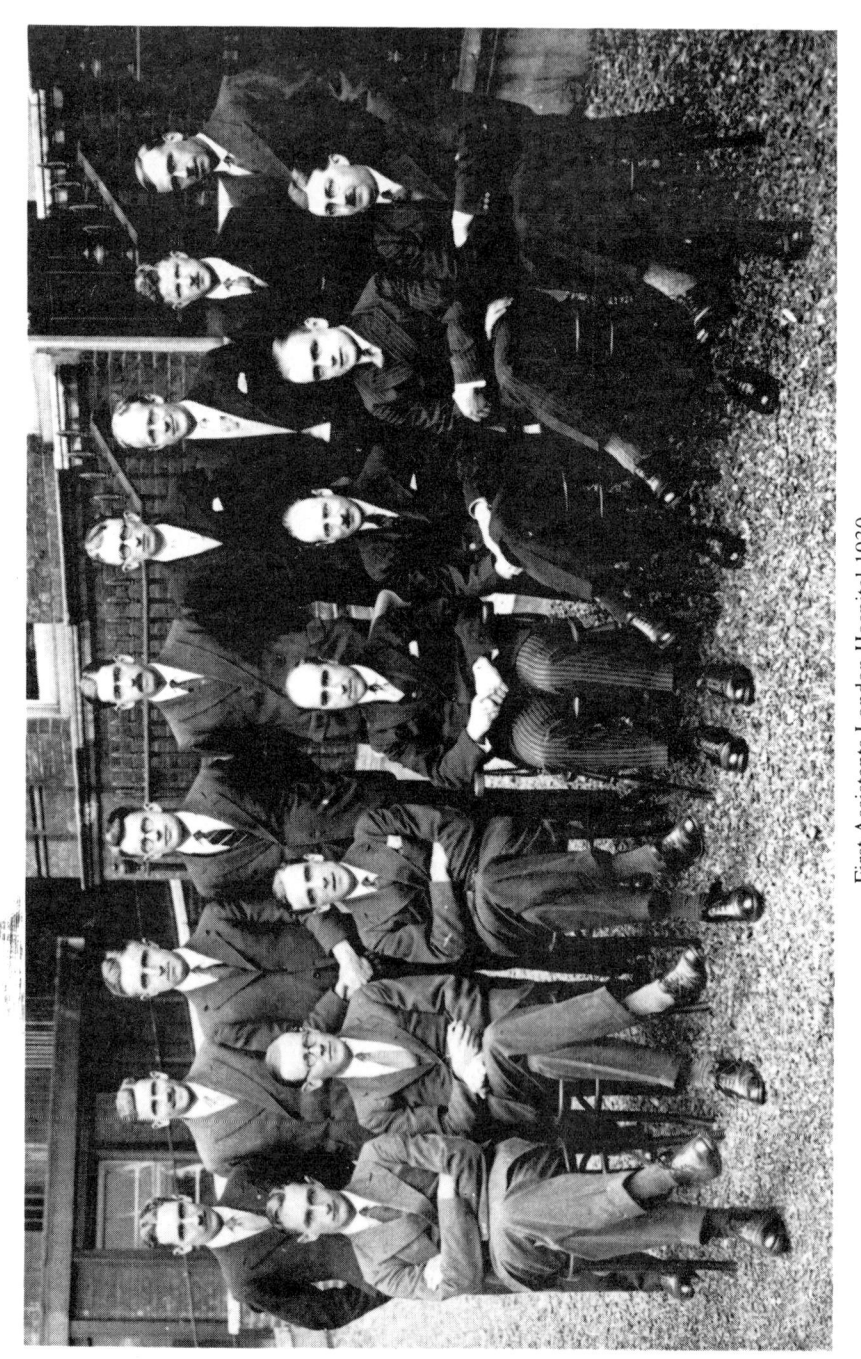

First Assistants London Hospital 1930.

S. H. Cookson, R. M. Bates, B. F. Russell, E. W. Skipper, Stanford Howard, Horace Evans, A. C. Gairdner, J. C. Hoyle, J. H. T. Challis, R. K. Debenham, F. B. Byrom, Charles Donald, R. T. Brain, K. H. Tallerman, R. A. Brews, William Evans.

*(Absent:* J. V. O'Sullivan)

*(Reproduced by kind permission of Mr J. Evans, The Royal London Hospital, Archives Dept.)*

April 1926 and withdrew his application in Cardiganshire on 22 January 1926. He spent most Sunday afternoons studying his records and slides. He had gained a Pathology Prize as a student writing an essay on 'Causes of Brain Abscess' and he regarded this post as one of the most important which he held. As he said 'the clinician has to search the truth from his patient, the pathologist has the stark truth before him'.

After that he became house physician to Dr John (later Sir) Parkinson who became the greatest influence on his life and inspired him to undertake research. On his first morning he was told that none of his patients was to have tablets or medicines, unless it was an emergency, until Dr John[9] had examined the patient. At the time he thought Dr John had no confidence in him but it made him realise how patients improved with rest and nursing care.

He was appointed Receiving Room Officer and Senior Medical and Surgical Assistant to the Outpatient Department from October 1927 to October 1930. He then became first Assistant and Medical Registrar (1930-33), Assistant Director of the Medical Unit July 1934-October 1935 and was appointed Assistant Physician to the Medical Department in July 1934. (Appx. III.) On the 15th June 1938 he was nominated Assistant Physician to the Cardiac Department at the Hospital; this department having an international reputation.

In 1944 he was appointed Physician to the National Heart Hospital. With the advent of the National Health Service in 1948 he became Consultant Physician to the Cardiac Department at the London Hospital, National Heart Hospital and Institute of Cardiology.

In December 1927 he gained the M.D. and in January 1928 the MRCP proceeding to FRCP in 1935.

He had gained the K.E.D. Payne Prize in Pathology in 1927, £20 for an essay on 'Pathology of Brain Abscess' and the Liddle Triennial Prize of £120 in Pathology in 1930 and £20 for an essay on 'The Cause and Incidence of Duodenal Ulcer' the first Welshman to gain this prize. These essays are in London Hospital College Library. In 1929 he received the Hutchinson Prize £60 for clinical Surgery. He was Paterson Research Scholar Oct. 1930-April 1933 getting £400 per year and a Research worker to the Medical Research Council 1933-1934. In 1946 he gained a D.Sc. in the University of London receiving it at the Royal Albert Hall on 2 May.

⁹ Minerva Obituary Dr John Parkinson by William Evans. *Br.Med.Jr.* 1976. 30 Oct. p. 1080.

William Wright, Dean of the London Hospital in his reference in 1926 wrote that WE had an unusually wide and varied experience of diseases of children as the London Hospital with its numerous children's wards meant it was the largest Children's Hospital in London. Dr John Parkinson in 1932 wrote that WE was the best House Physician he had had, and was a born teacher, experienced and self-critical in research and eminently suitable for an appointment on the staff of a teaching hospital. He was an experienced physician, of stirling character, cheerful temperament who did sound work. Theodore Thompson in 1930 wrote that he was an industrious worker who had a flair for original work.

He applied to become Physician to the Outpatient Department of the National Hospital for Diseases of the Heart. In his letter of the 20 November sent with his application he ends by telling them that 'should you honour me with the appointment I shall spare no effort to fill the post worthily'. His references at this time pay tribute to his great reputation as a teacher, being one of the most popular with students. Professor Arthur Ellis referred to him as charming, loyal, unselfish, having high ideals, careful and thorough in all his work, being a source of strength. Professor H. M. Turnbull refers to him as being a researcher by nature and finding in his clinical work a rich field for research. 'He works quickly, quietly and with great thoroughness'. While he was a Pathology Assistant in 1926 he analysed on his own initiative and without any help from the Directors, the cases of abscess of the brain in the hospital records from 1908 and for this work he was awarded the K.E.D. Payne Prize. This was published in the *Lancet* in 1931.

At the National Heart Hospital he expected all the niceties of protocol.[10] He would arrive dressed in striped trousers, spats, black coat and bowler hat. An assistant would be expected to greet him and take the bowler hat and woe betide him if he was not there. He would arrive at 1 p.m. to do a Ward round until 2 p.m. than a postgraduate teaching clinic for ten trainees followed by X-ray screening of the patients.

[10] Lewis, M. Personal Information.

Chapter 4

# Teaching, Lectures and Clinics

In a letter to the *Western Mail* on 'Welsh Greats', Byron Evans'[11] pointed out that until 1960 WE was the greatest teacher of Cardiology in the world, who had been asked to give lectures of distinction in the Commonwealth, Europe and America. Willie[12] thought there were two objectives to teaching medicine. The first was imparting academic and scientific knowledge with emphasis on basic principles, and the second the artistry of good doctoring. He was a master of the doctor patient relationship. He made a case for integration of preclinical and clinical studies which would bring fresh inspiration for the medical student. A knowledge of the Humanities was important in the art of healing and the ability to converse and discourse. Words were often better therapeutic agents than medicines. He never let medical students forget the need to support and sustain the sufferer and quoted Hippocrates often 'The Patient should never be worse off for seeing a doctor'.[13] He was always kind, sympathetic, and reassuring giving the truth in simple words.

Dr John H. Owen[14] of Porthcawl said he was precise and unequivocal who warned his students not to quote him in exams as they would fail! He made them take vows with him and all present had to bring out note books to write the vows down. One of his pet aversions was the term Mitral Incompetence. One vow was that 'In every case of Hypertension I shall feel for the femoral pulse' and another 'In a patient with Mitral Stenosis I shall have come to the diagnosis on clinical grounds before asking for a history of Rheumatic Fever.'

He was a didactic teacher 'write it down doctor, write it down'! His students all knew what he thought.

[11] Evans, B. Welsh Greats Correspondence, *Western Mail*, 9 Nov. 1981.
[12] Evans, W. Personal Papers.
[13] Evans W. Treatment of Cardiac Infarction BMA Toronto 1955.
[14] Owen, J. H. Feedback 'Evans-isms' Medikasset Vol. 17 No. 6 p. 18.

On teaching[15] he had an opinion as he did on everything else. He thought that the good teacher was born not made but that training helped to a certain extent. A lecture should not be impromptu and the lecturer should never be casual or ill-prepared.

A substantial sonorous vibrant voice was a help for the audience to enjoy and an erect, alert and upright posture commanded respect. This was enhanced if he stood on a platform and not on the floor when lecturing. In this he quoted his schooldays friend Dr Martyn Lloyd-Jones, a notable preacher who was ill at ease standing on the floor at a breakfast gathering and not addressing them from the pulpit. WE had himself written sermons and practised them in the barn when he was planning to follow Divinity at Lampeter.

He did not think that there were set rules for teaching other than a thorough knowledge of the subject to be imparted but the method the teacher used should be his own with the use of aids. A testimony of a student was 'He holds my attention. I understand what he says. He convinces me that what he says is true. I can remember the things he has said'. Another American Student was heard to say 'Gee! if that guy ever came to America we would make him President of the United States.'

Educationalists say that teachers should not spoon feed their pupils but encourage them to think for themselves and find out things for themselves but he encouraged his students to take vows with him and repeat them.

He once met an old student[16] in the lift of the Royal Society of Medicine (RSM) and asked whether she had a recollection of anything he said which she thought worth remembering. She replied immediately 'yes – you said that no patient should be worse for seeing a doctor. You called on me to take a vow that I should remember it and practice it. I did and I do'. He had an unique ability to convey a message and came alive in the consulting room like a great performer, using his hands with Welsh 'Hwyl'.

'A good teacher should not weary the student but should guide and instruct and imbue him with a spirit of adventure which will lead to proficiency and perfection. Medicine used to be an art, today it is not all science but a complex calling'.

He lectured world wide and lists 64 places where he was invited but this did not include Rhyl where he gave the first Winkup Lecture in the

15 Evans, W. Personal Papers.
16 Cooke, B. Personal Correspondence.

new postgraduate centre in the Royal Alexandra Hospital on 26 November 1970 on 'Old truths exemplified anew'. He also delivered 10 Memorial Lectureships which gave him great satisfaction. (Appx. IV.)

The first European Congress of Cardiology was held in London in September 1952 organised by The British Cardiac Society with Sir John Parkinson as Chairman. WE spoke on 'The Electrocardiogram of Cardiac Pain' giving his results on 1000 consequtive patients with cardiac pain.

On the opening day he entertained foreign guests to lunch at Frascati's Restaurant.

At the first International Congress of Cardiology in Paris the talks could not begin in any of the five separate theatres because no lanterns were working. When his turn arrived the lantern was working but no pointer was available so he impoverished with a rolled up newspaper. By the second day all faults had been corrected.

When the 2nd International Congress took place in Washington four years later, no suitable lantern was available to project his $3^{1}/_{4}''$ x $3^{1}/_{4}''$ slides although he had asked for this facility two months earlier. He asked for a blackboard but one could not be found which gave him cause for comment before his talk that facilities available in the Old World were missing in the New.

In 1954 after speaking at this 2nd International Congress of Cardiology in Washington on 'Early ECG signs of Coronary Heart Disease' he carried out a Lecture Tour of Maryland, Philadelphia, McGill, Rochester, Evanston and Cleveland.

He was invited to give the Gerrish Milliken Memorial Lecture in Philadelphia. The Chairman had told him that he wanted to attend a closed-circuit television session in another part of the City following his talk when a film on treatment of high blood pressure was being shown. As he walked to the rostrum the Chairman whispered he hoped that he would not speak for too long. Half way through the Chairman appeared at his side, apologised, gave him 100 dollars and took him to the other meeting where he had to listen to high praise being given to a drug he had earlier been denigrating. A memorable memorial lecture for which he was generously recompensed for saying so little.

A lecture he gave on an aspect of coronary artery disease at a congress in a remote hospital in Italy[17] when he was representing Great

[17] Congress in Italy 1956.

21

Britain was relayed to the Vatican and when he had an audience with the Pope later his Holiness reviewed the subject matter discussed at the Conference. During the Congress the use to which this remote centre could be put were discussed and Paul White's (who was representing the U.S.A.) idea was that it should become a centre for the study of psychosomatic disease which found favour with the Pope.

On being asked how many people worked in the Vatican, Pope John replied 'About a half'!

WE found the Conference a moving occasion for the idea for the hospital was that of a humble saintly parish priest who had received the stigmata on his hands and feet of the wounds made by the nails that held Christ to the Cross. Over the years Padre Pio had been visited by pilgrims who had come for his blessing and gave him gifts which had made him wealthy and with this he decided to build a hospital. This man had given up worldly comfort to serve his fellow man.

On May 2nd 1999 the Pope, in what the *Times*[18] called one of the most spectacular acts of his 21 year reign, put Padre Pio, the controversial mystic friar and faith healer, on the road to Sainthood before an audience of more than half a million as one of the 'Saints for the new Millennium'.

He died in 1968 at the age of 81. He is the first priest acknowledged by the Vatican to have borne stigmata since St. Francis of Assisi in 13 century. The Pope presided over the Beatification ceremony which is the step before Canonisation.

WE was a resourceful man who was well prepared always and at one lecture he was to give in Ireland[19] visited the Hall the day before and found there were no facilities to darken it but this task was delegated to the priest; the slide projector was ancient and had no plug and he had to use his nail file as a screw-driver and his manicure scissors was also needed with the flex. The white screen was so delicate that it was decided to erect it when everyone was in place. A bamboo stick was used as a pointer and for a lectern a golden eagle with spread out wings was procured from the church.

The proceedings the following day started late but all went well and in the early hours of the following morning he proposed the toast to 'The Guests' having been asked to do so at the dinner!

[18] Owen, R. 'The Pope puts mystic on road to Sainthood' *The Times*, May 3, 1990, p. 14.
[19] Evans, W. 'Whither Cardiology?' Jr. Roy. Col.Surg. Ireland 1963, Vol. 1, No. 1, p. 13-27, 1st Leonard Abrahamson Memorial Lecture.

In January 1955 he had a hemicolectomy but this did not prevent him continuing lecture tours and in 1958 visiting Copenhagen[20] to speak at a World Health Organisation meeting on the action needed to curb diseases of the heart and blood vessels. Twelve leading specialists from ten countries met and the two invited from Britain were WE and Dr J. N. Morris. This was at a time when infectious diseases were being conquered but the death rate from heart diseases was rising and was higher in Britain than in the Netherlands.

He gave his Stethoscope[21] to a local Tregaron boy who went in for medicine and on telling one of his teachers whose it was, was given the advice, 'I should treasure that'.

When he was ninety, Minerva in the BMJ[22] remembered him with affection and almost with awe on behalf of generations of students to whom he taught cardiology. Minerva also remembered his compassion and his emphasis on the importance of a good education for socially deprived children with rheumatic heart disease who would be ill-suited to manual work.

At his eightieth birthday party in Cardiff on November 29, 1975 an album from his friends was given to him as thanks for the courtesy, help and kindness he had given them during many years of valued friendship.

Frederic Jackson wrote that the vows had not been forgotten but greater than this was the example he had given of how to be a true doctor. George Kiloh was a friend whose name appeared often in the five year diary and who had written 'Lives of great men all remind us we can make our lives sublime and departing leave behind us footprints on the sands of time'.

Some general quotes he left were:–

'No one should write a book unless he has a message to convey, too many books are messageless'.

'To be dumb at a patients bedside is to miss the opportunity to make him better'.

'Euthanasia is murder glossed over'.

'Artistry should be part of instruction and communication'.

'Better health than wealth' which he had as a motto on his crest as High Sheriff.

[20] Heart Disease Campaign, *Daily Telegraph*, 17 April 1958.
[21] Evans Frances – Personal Communication.
[22] Minerva – William Evans, 90 – *Brit.Med.Jr.* 1985 291.1583.

On Humour he wrote that English terminology is not free from ambiguity and gave as an example a Chairman of a medical gathering in Montreal introducing him to the audience saying 'Those of you who have not enjoyed listening to William Evans before, will hear him now!'

He had great fun at a BMA Lecture[23] telling his audience he was in a bit of a dilemma. He wondered whether he was an interloper, a gate-crasher at the table and gracious hospitality that evening. Was the invitation meant for someone else?

First, the letter had been addressed to the 'The Consulting Physician to the Cardiff Department of the London Hospital.' When he retired from the London's Cardiac Department there was no Cardiff Department in the hospital. 'It may have been founded there since by my friend Dr Byron Evans, for let me add that at the London Hospital, Byron and Cardiff mean the same thing.'

Next, the letter was directed to Tregarne. He lived in Tregaron, 'but the Welsh Language Society may have changed the name unbeknown to me'. 'Thirdly, I was apostrophised as 'Dear Sir William'. 'Certainly I have neither the claim nor merit to that distinction.'

'Fourthly I deciphered the signature as Alun Williams, so I feared I was being inveigled into the arms of the B.B.C. which God forbid!'

When flying to Egypt[24] Dr Evans was told by the air hostess that he might be interested to know that Errol Flyn was seated behind him. Dr E. answered 'Tell Mr Flyn that Dr William Evans is seated just in front of him'.

*Recreation*

In the 135th Annual Meeting of the BMA in Bristol in 1967[25] he points out the need for doctors to have a knowledge of the Humanities, Classics, Communication and a need for integration of Clinical and non Clinical teaching e.g. in endocrine disease; histology and arrhythmias. There was need for close contact with patients. A need for renewing, refreshing and refurbishing medicine, and better student selection. A need for adequate time for good doctoring and he felt the NHS did not allow for this.

*Private Practice*

He had a thriving private practice which included foreign Royalty, National and International figures, who visited him in Harley Street.

[23] Evans, W. BMA Lecture Cardiff. 1972. Personal Papers.
[24] Cooke, B. Personal Correspondence.
[25] Recreation. 135th Annual Meeting BMA Bristol July 13 1967.

He was also asked to go abroad e.g. in 1950 he was asked to go to Kuwait to see the Ruler, but preferred seeing them in London where he had all the latest facilities at hand. On one occasion he was flown to Paris for a consultation but was back in London in time for his Clinic.

Although he received £25 honorarium per year for teaching at the London Hospital his fees were dependent on private practice in 15 Harley Street. This house had been owned by Thomas Johnes of Hafod, Cardiganshire whose daughter Marianne died there.

Joan Cooper[26] was his private secretary for four years and recalls at her interview a portly serious man formally dressed standing in a sombre consulting room dominated by a vast oil painting of a sailing ship buffeted by a huge sea of storm swept waves. She suggested later that flowers be placed in the consulting room to help soften the atmosphere and he agreed with this. Two days were spent in hospital and three in private practice but all patients were treated in the same manner. He allowed her to completely organise his office and enjoyed his confidence and cooperation. The administration of his files was simple and methodical and he would either dictate to her or write in his legible tidy handwriting for her type.

Before Christmas 1955 he had not been well but as he did not want to upset his family, had done nothing about it until after the Festival. He asked her to ring Mr Ivor Griffiths and she asked him 'Which Patient'? He replied 'Me'!

He sent the surgeon a bottle of champagne every year he survived – until the surgeon died! He was strong and healthy. 'Do what I say and not what I do' was one of his favourite sayings.

After she married she could not continue the long hours working for him but that period of her life was one of the most enjoyable.

After his wife died he would visit her family for Sunday lunch and helped to keep her boys entertained by encouraging them to long jump. Without moving from his chair he instructed them to find two long sticks and lay them parallel on the lawn about 18 inches apart. Then they had to jump across them and when they could clear them, then and only then could they be placed further apart. A simple expedient that kept them well entertained and developed their athletic abilities.

They visited him for holidays in Bryndomen and his death left a great hole in their lives as he had taken such an interest in their children and grandchildren. Although he refused television in his home

[26] Cooper, J. M. – Personal Correspondence.

in the 70's when the family were competing in 'Ask the Family' he would watch their weekly appearance on the TV Set at Tyndomen, writing afterwards to cheer them on to the next round.

He was a good trencherman and wrote profusely to thank her for the annual Christmas cake she sent him.

She found him modest, kindly and highly intelligent; thoughtful and considerate of others whilst holding definite clear views and high principles about life. It had been a great privilege for her to have known and worked for such a remarkable man.

He wrote a most delightful appreciative letter of thanks[27] to a patient who had brought him a gift in Harley Street in 1967 which can stand as a testament to him.

'I have just halted for a tea-break and I dipped into the box which you so kindly laid on my table this morning. I have tasted and tested Welsh-cakes this world over (for I have had them in America) including Wales, and at the hands of diverse cooks, among them my Niece, a domestic science teacher at Tregaron County School, but none has been so delicious as these. They really are delicious and while thanking you for your most kind thought, I also congratulate you on your culinary skill'.

It is charming and fulsome in its praise of the Welsh-cake but also shows his literary accomplishment.

*Clinics*

His clinics were memorable. Besides undergraduates there were always a few postgraduate students from other hospitals present at the London. Dr Evans examined a patient himself first and then asked about five students to listen to the heart sounds. On occasion he would ask those who had heard the first heart sound to raise their hand and likewise the second, the third and fourth sounds. His teaching was along basic principles.

Professor Brian Cooke[28] remembers a patient who had recovered from two coronaries asking Dr Evans if he could make a visit away from home. Dr Evans readily agreed and when the patient left he was asked why he had done so, since it seemed that the patient would have another coronary which could prove fatal. His answer was, that if the patient only had a short time to live, then it was better he should do

[27] Simon C. – Collection File No. 4. 26 July 1967. National Library of Wales.
[28] Cooke, B. – Personal Correspondence.

what he wished, than be restricted to his home and treated as an invalid. That was around 1941 when medical and surgical treatment available was minimal compared to that today.

Dr Evans explained that when he saw someone in the street with a basal cell carcinoma on the face he would give the patient his card and tell him to contact his G.P. He did this with several patients for varying spot diagnosis especially of Thyroid disease. This was 'Wayside Doctoring' for the highly skilled only.[29] One lady to whom he gave a peppermint in Princes Street, Edinburgh for the relief of pain was told she had flatulent dyspepsia, not angina, and didn't need amyl nitrate.

In the 1940's classes were not as large as they are today and Dr Evans knew everyone by name. He remembered Prof. Cooke and his wife a former nurse at the London by name when they met him over breakfast at the RSM years later.

He was a giant among many giants such as Russell Howard, Sir Horace Evans, Sir John Parkinson, George Riddock, Turnbull, Clarke Kennedy etc. He had no visual aids only chalk and a blackboard and handouts were almost non existent. Most successful teachers were extroverts and actors, and often it was their personal magnetism and charisma that made their clinics and lectures so memorable and enjoyable. WE was superb at this and developed his own style and mannerisms.

John H. Owen[30] remembered an international gathering of cardiologists one day in the clinic who were asked 'Why don't you get a presystolic murmur in the presence of Atrial fibrillation?' All sorts of theories were put forward and then WE asked JHO to give the correct answer.

(JHO) 'Because Sir James McKenzie said so.'

(WE) 'Stand up and face the congregation.'

'This little chap writing home to his mother can say he has beaten this gathering – he is clerk on my firm, his memory is only a week old – sit down!'

When JHO was sitting the conjoint exam after he had given his findings in the clinical he was asked,

'Did you not expect a presystolic murmur?'

'No', he proudly replied.

'Why not?'

[29] Taylor of Harlow, 'Wayside Doctor'. Personal View. *Brit.Med.Jr.* 1976. ii. 392.
[30] Owen, J. H. – 'Evans-isms'. Medikasset. Vol. 17, No. 6, p. 18.

Pavlovian response, 'Because Sir James McKenzie said so'.
Examiner 'and so have others'.
He passed!'

There were no women students in his day. The men always dressed neatly in suits or blazer and Daks and always wore a tie. Nobody had long hair or beards.

Ex-Service students after the War were well received. Some were married while before the War there were no married students. 'Dr W. Evans' warm, friendly outgoing personality shone as an example to us all, as how the ideal physician should relate to his patients and students.'

Dr Malcolm Towers[31] remembers his enthusiasm for the London Hospital, which he pronounced 'Lunnon Hospl', and Cardiology; his immense and unfailing support for young people and the advances he was able to make in Cardiology, which then was a physics based subject, through native shrewdness and with little knowledge of basic science.

He was a man of his time. Patients and medical students were always addressed by their surnames and Consultants (though not WE) could be exceedingly rude to both.

There was no counselling: people had misfortunes (their friends would try and support them) and they had to get on with things. Doctors were held in much higher esteem than Doctors today though they could do infinitely less for patients.

Because comparatively little was known scientifically the personality of the doctor was all important.

He was very proud of the London and the Cardiac Department – one of the top departments in probably the top teaching hospital at that time. Students were always being invited to gaze at the photograph of Sir James McKenzie and many of his young men went on to senior and top jobs in Cardiology. If you had worked for him and applied for a job elsewhere he would find out who was on the appointments Committee and each member telephoned in turn and told whom to appoint! Some of his staff were always, even to the last years, slightly in awe of him and though most regarded him as 'Willie', 'Sir' was the usual form of address.

WE was an enthusiast for Fluoroscopy.

He was interested in Triple Rhythm when MT was there and this led him into Phonocardiography using a double string galvanometer.

---

[31] Towers, M. Personal Communication.

28

John Parkinson had brought Aubrey Leatham into the department and WE took him over to advance Phonocardiography. With the help of Joe Spencer (of Cardiac Recorders) AL made great advances and with MT's interest in physics and electronics he followed him. They were heady times – it seemed something new and important would be discovered almost every week! AL and to a lesser extent MT went on to study the behaviour of the second heart sound. WE attached great importance to the naming of new discoveries – 'ejection murmurs', 'pan systolic murmurs' etc. – his team would sit for hours (it seemed) working on it. MT thought it all rather a bore, 'we knew what he meant'. Every time MT hears the term 'partial prolapse of one of the mitral cusps' – a name which is scientifically correct but for a trivial condition sounds horrendous to patients – he thinks of WE – he would never have allowed it!

When a new advance burst upon the scene WE would have a definite opinion almost at once. 'Cardiac catheterisation – it would never catch on'. Anticoagulants for coronary disease – 'rat poison'. On hearing in 1974 that they had gone out of favour he observed 'Someone tried hard to stop them coming in twenty years before!'

He was largely but not totally right that time. He demanded the highest standards in records of all kinds – ECG, phonocardiograms and photographs of X-rays for his books and publications. If they were less than perfect his faithful technician the late Bill Dicks would have to repeat them. He was a founder member and President of the Society of Cardiological Technicians in 1948 which still prospers 50 years on.

He was a didactic teacher 'write it down Doctor, write it down'. His aphorisms are written in a book which Frances has. All his students knew what he thought. There were countless stories of WE some of which he told against himself. A newly appointed Senior Registrar had resolved to civilise the department. He arranged for coffee to be served in the department in the middle of the morning and Willie was taken aback. There was a visitor who had been Babinski's houseman present. 'Did Babinski stop for coffee?' WE asked. I do not think that the visitor understood the question for he faltered 'There you see' said WE 'Babinski never stopped for coffee' and that was that!

The students were taught in quite a large room – say 25ft x 25ft and sat in four or five rows. A patient would be brought in, a history taken and then he was examined on a couch. The students would be asked questions during this period. One patient, as he left said 'I met your bruvver Sir 'Orace yesterday' (Sir Horace later Lord Evans). Rumour had it that there was no love lost between the two Dr Evans. The door was shut behind the patient and the class waited for the explosion. 'Never to refuse a complement however oblique' said WE!

An article by Eirian (Bill) Williams[32] in the BMJ captures the outpatient scene beautifully.

WE used to teach that reassurance is the most precious pill which we have at our disposal. He coined the aphorism 'It is better to do nothing than something, when nothing needs to be done'.

Also, 'among the many medicaments which doctors carry in their bags, there can be none more precious than Reassurance,[33] precious in that it is the 'pill' he has to dispense most frequently and so often does most good'.

Age is an advantage when giving an opinion and as he said 'Age buys experience and in medicine, experience is a precious commodity'.

He also taught that it is important not to qualify reassurance. If the patient is normal no qualification is necessary and he deplored doctors indecisiveness in qualifying an opinion so that a patient is not reassured after the consultation. He described the placebo[34] effect and to get the full effect from it, advice needs to be given enthusiastically. He said that no patient should be the worse for seeing a doctor.

He had an understanding of why patients wanted to leave hospital even if this could damage their health. The boredom, noise, discipline, food, lack of privacy and depression as well as the disease and its treatment make them want to escape. A student[35] told WE that the patient he was examining wished to take his own discharge. 'Why do you think he wants to do that? asked WE. 'I have no idea Sir' the student replied 'we have hardly begun his treatment'. WE turned to the Registrar and said 'Make sure this student is warded before he qualifies'.

He had a serious illness and was twice an inpatient and said 'Every doctor should welcome incarceration in a hospital bed for a short time. Not till then will his medical education be complete'.

David Mendel has said 'it is a virtuoso performance, humanity and wit which makes men into giants. It is not the projected image but the

[32] Williams, E. Chance, Coincidence, Serendipity – The biter bit. Brit.Med. Jr. 1980. 281. 1190.
[33] Mendel, D. Proper Doctoring. Springer-Verlag 1984 p. 134, 135.
[34] Evans, W. & Hoyle C. 'The Comparative Value of Drugs used in the continuous treatment of Angina Pectoris'. *Quart. J. Med.*, 1933, 26, 311.
[35] Mendel, D. Personal Communication.

polished skills as performers which make them first rate. He hero worshipped WE, who was superior, tall, portly and avuncular with a soft Welsh voice and good manners. He liked him more than any other cardiologist of his day because he was a "gent", used gentle persuasion and had a high comedy wit'.

Although he worked very hard he never appeared too busy. He recorded everything and wrote with clear hand writing. He was a careful observer. measured and recorded scientific date but did not bother much with statistics or biophysics. If he liked a treatment he would use it. He used his loaf!!

One of his favourite tricks was to diagnose people in the street, go up to them, hand them his visiting card and tell them to show it to their doctor. On the back was written 'doctor, your patient is suffering from . . .' often this was Thyroid disease. The patients were delighted but the doctor who had missed the diagnosis would have mixed feelings!

Once when WE went to visit the London Hospital on a Sunday there was a long queue of patients' visitors. Willie walked to the top of the queue and the porter said 'Back of the queue mate' to which Willie replied 'I am a consultant here' to which the porter replied 'Don't make no difference mate, back of the queue', and then Willie said: 'But my wife is a Ward Sister here' to which the porter replied: 'Why didn't you say so, in you go'. Willie told David Mendel this with great joy.

MT said that WE always expected high standards of his staff. Diagnosis was all important as there was so little treatment and tests could take all afternoon. He expected everything to be perfect for photographic records of Phonocardiography and Bill Dicks his technician would have to repeat everything if they were not to his satisfaction. The patient was expected to breathe in and out for the photographic plates and this could be difficult as the timing of the murmurs was important and WE was interested in heart sounds. This vogue for Phonocardiography lasted 10 years and then Paul Wood took over cardiac catherisation which WE thought a fad which would not last!

WE was of an era where men were addressed by their Surname and I saw a letter written by him to MT in 1985 with the same neat and tidy handwriting 'Dear Towers' yet signed off 'William'. As MT said 'He must have known my Christian name well as my friends used it'.

He saw private patients in Harley Street and in 1952 my childhood friend Sheila[36] who was a 2nd MB Medical Student in Kings at the time

---

[36] Cross, S. R. Personal Communication.

took her father there to see him. WE admitted him immediately to the National Hospital and in three days he was dead from Aortic Stenosis. Sheila had met her Father in Paddington and found he was very breathless. His General Practitioner had decided to send him to London to see Dr William Evans. They went straight to Harley Street and were seen in a dark back room. He showed Sheila the ECG and pointed out inverted T waves but she had never seen an ECG previously and had no idea what it meant. He was not patronizing in any way but she did not ask him the significance of the ECG and on her return to Kings went to see one of her lecturers to ask what it meant. WE took the trouble to write her a very nice letter which unfortunately is not available now and told her he could not tell her how ill her father was at the time and that if she needed help with her career she was to get in touch with him. He did not charge a fee for the consultation as her father was a Welsh Clergyman – a tradition which has now passed.

I heard from others too of his great kindness to his staff who were looking for appointments to further their career and he would personally telephone everyone he thought could help to impress on them the importance of appointing his candidate. This was one reason to command the loyalty of those who had worked with him.

Not everyone liked his style though – some found him unbearable because he was so didactic. others thought him pompous.

He would not use V leads on ECG and thought Limb leads best. He used three Limb leads and an inverted T wave in III he said was normal.

On one occasion when Willie was doing his usual trick of making the post-graduates at the National Heart Hospital (NHH) write things down an older doctor did not attempt to get his pen and paper out. 'Come along Doctor' said Willie 'You are not too old to learn!'

Another favourite trick was to get the postgraduates to try a Trinitrin. One Swiss lad was reluctant, took the pill and fell flat on the floor.

WE once looked at the X-ray of a man he wanted to reassure – one of his most usual ploys – and the heart was rather large due to Aortic Stenosis and Aortic Incompetence. 'You have got a heart like a bull' he said to the delighted man, and then turned to the staff and said 'Cor Bovinum' – a very serious condition.

By the time of his last outpatient clinic at the National Heart Hospital the audience he had been attracting was down to two or three

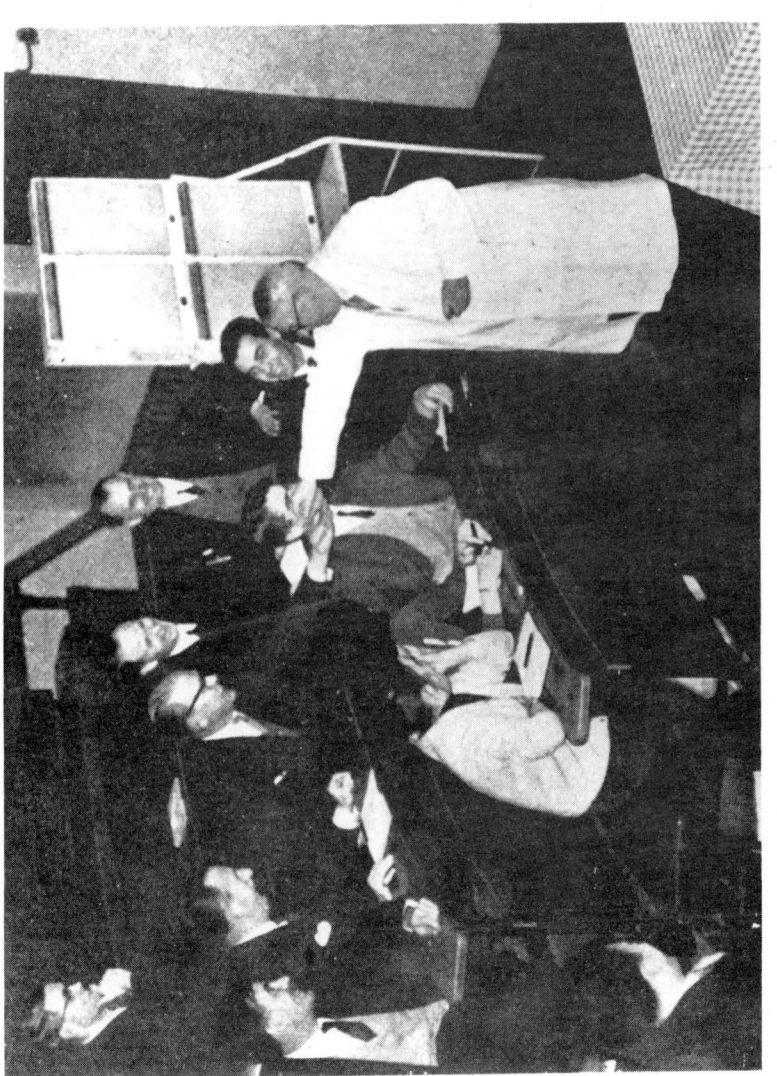

Dr Evans' final teaching round with poem he recited.

*(Reproduced by kind permission of Mr J. Evans, The Royal London Hospital, Archives Dept.)*

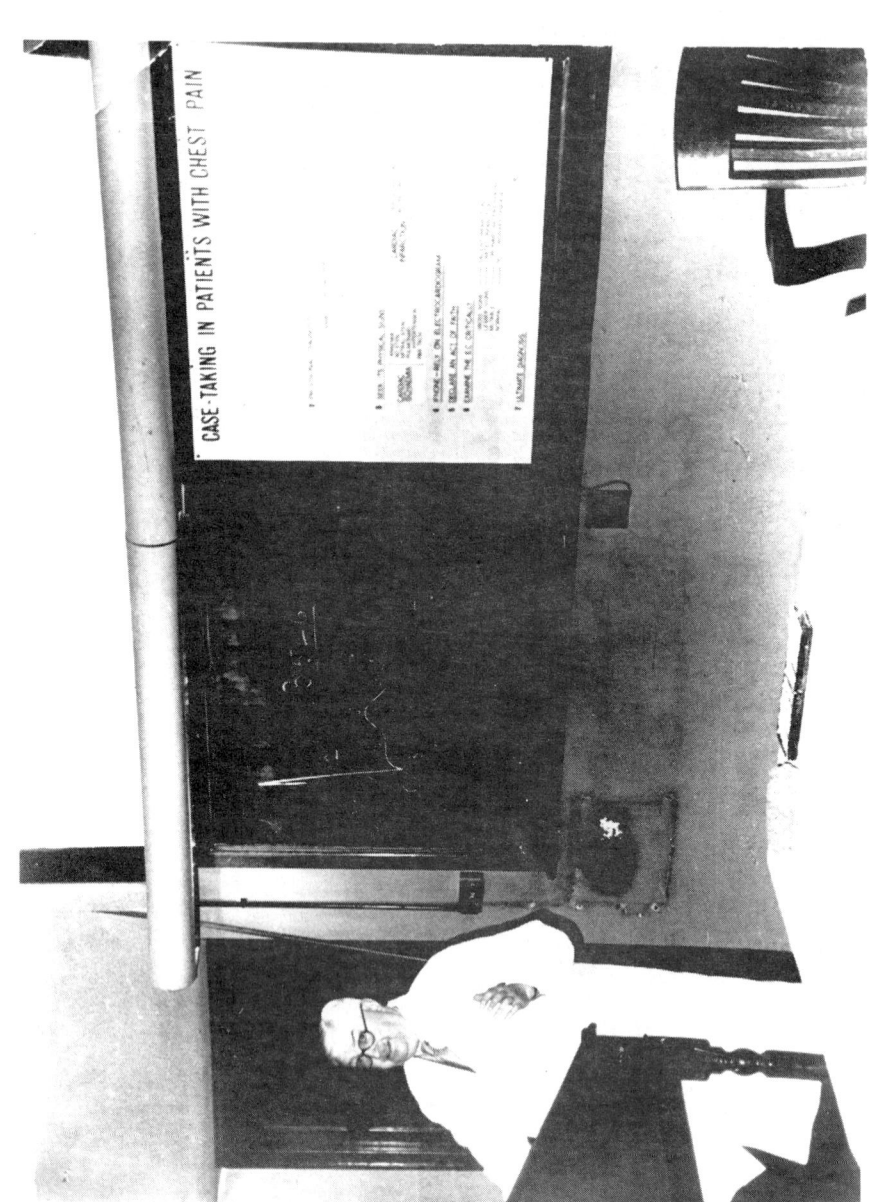

Dr Evans teaching.

(*Reproduced by kind permission of Mr J. Evans, The Royal London Hospital, Archives Dept.*)

post-graduates. Nothing had been laid on by the powers that be to celebrate his going and David Mendel[37] decided to make a fiesta of it. He wrote to all his past Registrars all over the world inviting them to the two o'clock clinic, to be followed by tea, for which he bought splendid cakes from Sagne's, one of London's best patisseries. Willie came at two and there were the usual three aficionados, and after about 10 minutes, Walter Somerville tiptoed in. 'Hello Walter, what are you doing here' said Willie. Walter replied 'Oh just passing Sir'. In the next hour about forty people came in, several from Wales and one from further afield.

At this point Willie's eye moistened but he just restrained himself. Over the course of the afternoon, his old confidence came back and he indulged in all his favourite cardiologist bating stories and these by now senior men argued happily with him, applauding at the appropriate moment. One of the Welsh (Byron Evans) had brought an iced cake with a Welsh inscription made by his wife. They all had a whale of a time. The hospital photographer came and took photographs which typically did not come out! Willie was tickled pink and very grateful.

David Mendel had never before or since organised a party for anyone and it is one of his happiest memories.

---

[37] Mendel, D. – Personal Correspondence.

Chapter 5

# Medical Books and Papers

Looking back over 40 years in Cardiology for the Sir Thomas and Lady Dixon Lecture in Belfast in 1965[38] he said that 'Cardiology seeped into my blood 40 years ago when I sat at the feet of Sir John Parkinson in the Cardiac Department of the London, which was the first Institute of its kind anywhere to direct its activities exclusively to the study of heart disease'.

He points out that during this time there have been many changes in terminology with some being discarded and some not. 'There is a need for more weeding and indeed for more planting, but any change must remain faithful to the principle that the newer version should convey a correct physiological and pathological interpretation'. He gives examples such as Auscultation Gallup rhythm becoming Triple Rhythm.

He makes a case for simple not complicated expressions. He did not believe in the habit of grading from 1-6 everything from heart disease to baldness and made a plea for uniformity in bedside terminology.

By the middle 30's he had published thirteen articles on Cardiovascular disease and eight on other subjects which included Anaemia of Pregnancy, postoperative gastric acidity, Banti's syndrome, Gaucher's Disease after Splenectomy, intrasacral epidural injection in the treatment of Sciatica, Duodenal Ulcer, Brain Abscess and Suppuration of the Lungs. During his lifetime he published more papers on cardiology than any other Cardiologist anywhere, 41 of them in the *British Heart Journal*.

He wrote classic papers on Congenital Coarctation of the Aorta, the Electrocardiogram in Friedreich's Disease, the heart in Myotonia Atrophica, Familial Cardiomegaly and Alcoholic Myocardiopathy which showed his knowledge of Medicine and of his ability to observe

---

[38] Evans, W. 'Forty Years in Cardiology' – Sir Thomas & Lady Dixon Lecture 12 October 1965. *Ulster Medical Journal,* Dec. 1965.

and record his findings. He could be provocative and controversial but had the ability to convey a message with common sense and sincerity. He gave several lectureships which are listed in Appendix V and he received the Sydney Body Gold Medal in Cardiology in 1954.

He undertook research on early diagnosis of coronary arterial disease through electrocardiography, the pathogenesis of systemic and pulmonary hypertension and clinical phonocardiography and admitted that chance often showed its hand.

The first electrocardiogram in man was carried out by Augustus Desiré Waller in 1887 using a Lippman capillary electrometer. The technique was impracticable for clinical use but it led to the introduction by Einthoven of his string galvanometer for clinical use in 1901. He selected the Cambridge Scientific Instrument Company of England as the original manufacturer. Much of the early work on the interpretation of electrocardiograms was carried out by Dr Thomas Lewis in University College Hospital London whose researches in this field ended in 1923 though W. H. Craib continued to carry out electrocardiography in his laboratory for another couple of years. Sir Thomas took little direct interest in this work and it came to a halt when Craib had disagreements with a number of notable authorities such as Lord Adrian.

Drury[39] gave two reasons why Lewis gave it up. Firstly it is suggested he grew tired of tackling questions the instruments could answer. He thought a problem should not be taken up unless it could be carried through. He also believed that if one had the capacity 'one should try and skim the cream off the milk and leave the skim to the others'. Lewis comments suggest that at 43 he had become tired of being tied to an elaborate instrument and that he had come to his natural end of studies on the disordered action of the heart. Hollman thought WE had overlooked the fact that straight forward observation was not Lewis' idea of progress in Medicine. Progress came from using the experimental method.

Lewis had never explored the importance of electrocardiography in the study of ischaemic disease and WE took an interest in it at this point.

'There is no future in this – I am giving it up' Lewis said to which WE replied 'Well in that case, I am taking it up'.

---

[39] Hollman, A. Sir Thomas Lewis, Springer 1996, p. 118.

When the Cardiac Society was first established the ECG was either hospital based or used in the consulting room. The development of portable apparatus enabled it to be taken into the patients home though at first this was impracticable as the photographic records needed developing in a dark room though with some machines this could be done on the spot. The first direct writing units only became widely used from 1950 onwards.

He found that the ECG may show signs of cardiac disease before cardiac pain is a symptom and that it was useful in recognising myocardial disease. The ECG could be interpreted in different ways by different cardiologists and one student's[40] memory was of a young man who had had an ECG, who was told he had had a heart attack and who threw himself off Westminster Bridge and drowned. The following day WE read the ECG and pronounced it normal showing the different way it could be interpreted by different cardiologists.

He advocated not saying anything to the patient of some early signs of coronary artery disease such as an absent S Wave[41] in lead 1 and present in lead 2 & 3 as it is only limited to the flow of blood to a small sector of the myocardium and cannot be a prediction for the future.

Another patient[42] visited him because he was disturbed after being discharged from hospital. He had sought an explanation for his illness. The family doctor had called it thrombosis, the house physician a coronary, the Registrar a blocked heart vessel, the Consultant an infarct, a patient in the ward – part of your heart is dead, finishing with a Sister who had wisely said 'it is better not to ask'. With feeling he said 'I am muddled and can not sleep'. Is it not better to say 'you had a heart attack which has passed?'

*History of Medicine*

WE was interested in the History of Medicine and taught it to his students. His Schorstein Memorial Lecture[43] in 1961 was published in the *London Hospital Gazette*. He was especially thrilled that it was a Welshman who had brought the stethoscope to London Hospital.

---

[40] Abrahams, A. H. 'It depends' Medikasset Vol. 18 No. 1, p. 18.
[41] Evans, W. Significance of S waves in Limb Leads 11 & 111 of ECG. Brit. Heart Jr. 1966 Vol. XXVIII No. 6 p. 829-834.
[42] Evans, W. Journey to Harley Street – David Rendel Ltd., London. 1968.
[43] Evans, W. History of Medicine – Schorstein Memorial Lect. Lond. Hospital Gazette Supplement 1961 Vol. LXIV, No. 4, ii-xx.

Thomas Davies 1759-1839 a native of Carmarthenshire founded the Royal Hospital for Diseases of the Chest in 1814. This was the first of its kind in Europe. After contracting Tuberculosis he had gone to Montpellier to recuperate and then went to Paris to study under Laennec where he got his M.D. in 1912. He had returned to London with a Laennec stethoscope which he introduced at the London. He became an Assistant at the London Hospital in 1827 when he was 68 years old but never attained the title Physician.

Herbert Davies 1818-1885, his son, became an Assistant Physician in 1845 and continued his father's work with the stethoscope. They both condemned percussion of the heart and Herbert pronounced that a Venous Hum in the neck was innocent. A book 'On the circulation of blood through diseased hearts' in 1889 published by Herbert Davies' Son, Dr A. T. Davies, four years after his death showed him to have been one of the foremost physicians of his day.

Archibald Billing 1791-1881 was physician to London Hospital 1822-1845 and was the first professor of Medicine at London University. He published text books in 1831 and 1852 on mechanisms of the heart sounds.

Jonathan Pereira 1804-1853 was born in Portugal and was appointed Assistant Physician to London in 1841. He published 'The Elements of Materia Medica and Therapeutics' in 1854 giving a detailed account of Digitalis. He died aged 49 having contributed 95 articles to the Pharmaceutical Journals and being made a Fellow of the Royal Society in 1838.

Ernest Sansom 1838-1907 was the son of a Wiltshire farmer and wrote on Cardiology when there was no sphygmomanometer, ECG or X-rays to assist him but he used sound reasoning to get the diagnosis. He wrote two textbooks on Heart Disease in 1881 & 1892 giving physical signs and making observations on heart sounds and murmurs. He designed the Binaural Stethoscope used today. He also pointed out that alcohol damaged the heart.

H. G. Sutton 1836-1891 wrote on Cardiovascular Hypertrophy and the importance of listening to heart sounds on auscultation. Then followed the Mackenzie Period. Leonard Hill 1866-1952 and Harold Barnard 1868-1908 devised a simple sphygmomanometer for clinical use in 1897 which became the prototype of a modern oscillometer and were independent of Riva-Rocci 1896. They experimented with anaesthesia and its effect on the blood pressure showing gas and oxygen increased the pressure, with ether it remained constant, and with chloroform it fell rapidly.

Arthur Keith 1866-1955 and Martin Flack 1882-1931 examined sections of the heart to find the s-a node and conducting fibres in animals, birds, fish and man.

James Mackenzie 1853-1925 was a big man in every sense who inspired his staff and stood alone in his generation accomplishing so much without facilities but by careful and astute observations. He wrote ten books on Cardiology and designed a polygraph to register the venous pulse. He had started as a Chemist's apprentice and when he was 21 years old went to Edinburgh to study Medicine, qualifying four years later. He became a General Practitioner in Burnley for 28 years, moving to London in 1907 and appointed to the Honorary Medical Staff of the Cardiac Department, London Hospital following his interest in the death of a young pregnant woman with atrial fibrillation.

John Parkinson 1885-1976 became Sir James Mackenzie's Chief Assistant. He installed an X-ray machine in the Cardiac Department and carried out Radiocardiology of the heart and great vessels. He was a good writer and teacher and carried on the clinical tradition of research. The cardiac department at the London took a prominent part in Coronary research and Angina. The Cardiac Department was founded in 1911 and in WE's day was the best department in London. It moved into new premises in 1931 and it was unique in that it had clinical and research facilities in the same building.

*The Incomparable Electrocardiogram*

WE wrote that 'to operate the Cambridge String Electrocardiograph was a feat in itself. A powerful arc lamp generated unwanted heat and inefficient light, which was enough to fog the plate, but not enough to trace the moving fibre. When optimum favourable photographic conditions prevailed the fibre might snap and the patient alone was unfrustrated and with three limbs immersed in suitably warmed saline solution he gazed in wonder at this mammoth machine at work. We only recorded three limb leads and what happy days they were'.

When he was House Physician to Parkinson, Evan Bedford was Registrar and 'I shared with them the thrill of discussing abnormal tracings. Soon the apical chest lead was added and later the posterior axillary lead CR7. Unipolar leads VR, V1, VF have contributed no single advantage'. He thought limb leads best.

38

Forty years had passed since Sir Thomas Lewis said of ECG that he had the cream off the milk and went on to study ischaemia of the limbs. WE said that what remained was not skimmed milk and the study has been rewarding. The reward of pinpointing lesser faults of ECG is rewarding in giving a secure diagnosis of cardiac pain.

He published a 'Students Handbook of Clinical Electro-cardiography'[44] in 1934 at the request of graduates and post graduates who sought his help in the interpretation of electrocardiograms when preparing for qualification or higher examinations in Medicine. It was a hardback of 49 pages and 64 illustrations dedicated to Dr John Parkinson in grateful recognition of his teaching and encouragement. In it he showed how to read an ECG giving examples of normal and abnormal readings concentrating on rate, rhythm, length of P-R interval, deviation of the electrical axis, and the form of the P wave, QRS complex and T wave.

He published many papers on electrocardiography.

*Phonocardiography*

When he first became curious about the nature of Heart Sounds additionally to the 1st and 2nd heart sounds he looked around for something to record them. There was not a standard machine available so a make-shift electrical one was assembled on the Laboratory bench and the sounds from the heart were fed into a carbon microphone. This primitive instrument made it possible to identify four kinds of sounds. After this work was done the separate murmurs came under review.

'In Mackenzie's old room there had lain two brown-paper parcels and these I had carried into the new department and deposited them tidily under a Lab. bench'. When he eventually opened them he found to his chagrin that they harboured the material parts of a phonocardiograph which Mackenzie had acquired 19 years beforehand but which he had never unpacked. 'The lesson is that when entering to work in a new post, the first step to take is to become familiar with the equipment and facilities which it offers and if the lesson were extended, to know the old before proclaiming it anew as if it were new'.

'At that time when my experience of phonocardiography had impressed me with its great value in clinical cardiology, it caused great

---

[44] Evans, W. *A Students Handbook of Clinical Electrocardiography*. H. K. Lewis, London 1934.

surprise that Sir Thomas Lewis after recording the murmur of patent ductus arteriosis, had abandoned its pursuance in the case of other auscultatory signs and in this to have failed to appreciate the benefit which the science could bestow on cardiology. Indeed phonocardiography should find a prominent place in the training of every young aspirant in Cardiology for through its agency he will acquire auscultatory discipline, because during his apprenticeship he will test his clinical impression of a sound or murmur through reference to their recording'.

'The art of auscultation is to listen, not to hear. Listening is to be attentive and freed from any preconceived ideas. It is systematic self-catechism'. WE gave the example of Samuel Levine of Boston who listened to and analysed each sound in turn. Once in the War when a 'Doodle Bug' went over the hospital WE said 'Can you hear another heart sound?'[45]

Cardiography[46] was a hardback of 132 pages and 211 figures divided into two sections which went to two editions the second in 1954. Part 1 described Electrocardiography and Part 2 Phonocardiography. In this, records were registered by a 'string galvanometer and the movement photographed alongside the simultaneous ECG. This is not a routine test and has no value on its own but has proved indispensable in establishing a clinical classification for added heart sounds and solving problems of innocent and organic murmurs. Auricular sound commences recording at or towards the end of the P wave and ventricular sound starts in the R-S period and is superimposed on the last phase of the auricular sound'.

Cardioscopy[47] was published in 1952 as a hardback of 143 pages and again dedicated to Sir John Parkinson. Radiological examination of the heart gives knowledge of the shape of the heart. He describes the use of orthodiagraphy, teleradiography, cardioscopy, kymography, tomography and angiocardiography in various normal and abnormal heart and great vessel conditions and demonstrates them with 207 plates.

He demanded the highest standards in electrocardiography and radiology and was largely responsible for putting auscultation on a proper scientific basis. He recognised the importance of the technician and was joint founder and 1st President of the Society of Cardiac

[45] Cooke, B. Personal Correspondence.
[46] Evans, W. Cardiography, Butterworth Publications. 1954.
[47] Evans, W. Cardioscopy, Butterworth Med. Publ. 1952.

Technicians. His faithful technician, William Dicks, did the photographic work for his publications as well.

Cardiology also went to two Editions, the second published in 1956 and Diseases of the Heart and Arteries was published in 1964. (Appx. III)

All his books were well written with style, clarity and precision. He carried out careful meticulous research and writing up his results in clear handwriting presented no problems for him and he enjoyed doing it.

*Papers*

He wrote a classic paper with Clifford Hoyle[48] in 1933 on 'The Comparative Value of Drugs used in the Continuous Treatment of Angina Pectoris'. They tested 13 drugs and a placebo and only four were more effective than the placebo which was 15 grains of sodium bicarbonate in half an ounce of infusion of gentian, with or without the addition of a minim of Carmine solution. The four drugs were chloral hydrate, morphine, papaverine and phenacetin in that order of effectiveness. However 27% showed great improvement with placebo and 10.5% moderate improvement.

In a letter to the *Lancet*[49] in 1963 he congratulates Dr Sandler and colleagues on the investigation of glyceryl trinitrate (GTN). He and Hoyle in 1934 had concluded that GTN has the greatest value in preventing painful attacks of angina, when they instructed patients to crunch the tablet not take it sublingually. If Sandler had done that they might not have concluded it had no value in the relief of an attack as it was important to ensure that the patient knows how to use it. The dose was 1/100 of a grain: When the pain set in the tablet should be chewed or crunched, the number taken should be liberal not limited.[50] The innocent pulsation in the head which may follow needs to be explained beforehand; the safety of the tablet should receive emphasis; the benefit gained from its prophylatic use should be specially stressed – namely that the tablet taken in mouth should be allowed to dissolve, shortly before exercise which brings on the pain.

[48] Evans, W. and Hoyle, C. The Comparative Value of Drugs used in the continuous treatment of Angina Pectoris. Quart.J.Med., 1933, 26, 311-338.
[49] Evans, W. Correspondence – In praise of Glyceryl Trinitrate, *Lancet* 1963 20th June, p. 1424.
[50] Evans, W. 'On Giving & Taking Medicines' – *Lond. Hosp. Gazette.* May 1959 ii-viii.

The value of the drug has been known since Murrell introduced it in 1879 and patients should carry it in in the waistcoat pocket of each suit, snuff boxes etc. It has no competitor.

In a Lecture to Winchester Division[51] of the BMA in 1962, reprinted in the BMJ he spoke that there were signs that the control of medicines was passing out of the hands of the medical profession. The profession needed to control their making and testing, sponsor their reliability, stand surety for their safety, and supervise their distribution and dispensing.

He poses the question of how many drugs do we need? The eight drugs he would take to a desert island would be morphine, digitalis, quinine, aspirin, antacid, a multiservice antibiotic, insulin and GTN. He was concerned that the National Drug Bill was rising and that much of medicinal therapy is governed by commercial and financial, not scientific and humanitarian need. Many of the newer toxic drugs had side effects. The number of hypertensive drugs was increasing and they had side effects.

He made a case for trenchant amendments through Medical Education. The undergraduate should guard against 'Rep' pressure. He thought there should be a National Therapeutic Trials Tribunal which would not be difficult to achieve and would set the standard of Therapeutics with economy, efficiency and safety. A national scheme working with the Medical Research Council was needed to test a drug by controlled clinical trial before it went on the market.

WE and Clifford Hoyle were the first to use the controlled trial. Until that time, new treatments were administered to patients and the outcome attributed to the treatment. They realised that a patients' condition could change for psychological reasons not connected with the treatment and so they gave dummy tablets to an equal number of patients of similar age, sex, and severity of symptoms. In this way changes which were not related to the treatment could be allowed for. He coined the phrase 'The placebo effect' in the 30's and this is now mandatory in the estimation of the efficiency of all new treatments. He was influenced by Sir John Parkinson's dictum not to prescribe medicine until he had examined the patient and found that rest alone had improved the picture.

[51] Evans, W. 'Addiction to Medicines' Brit. Med. Jr. 1962 – Lecture to Winchester BMA. Vol. ii p. 722-725.

He quoted Sir Robert Hutchinson's prayer a lot. This he had uttered from a Lecture Theatre at the London.

'From inability to let well alone,
from too much zeal for the new,
and contempt for what is old,
from putting knowledge before wisdom,
science before art, and cleverness before commonsense,
from treating patients as cases,
and from making the cure of disease more grievous than its endurance,
Good Lord, deliver us.'

In the 50's he stood courageously almost alone against the medical establishment in rejecting anticoagulants as protection against coronary disease. On hearing in 1974 that they had gone out of favour he observed 'Someone tried hard to stop them coming in twenty years before.'[52]

A new drug should improve the disease or symptoms in most instances, should have an effect which is greater than a placebo, and should never produce injurious symptoms.

He many times spoke against addressing laity on medicine as there is a danger of hypochondriasis and the Radio and TV misinterpret facts. Following an operation he could not sleep until he thought of that 'delectable river Teifi and of his early fishing experience of hazel rod, twine and bent pin and of the characters who taught him the art of fishing'.

He called his Wiltshire Memorial Lecture of 1961[53] 'To tell Trash from Treasure' and said the title had the smell of the market place about it. We are not unlike shopkeepers with patients as customers but the way we deal with health and the basis of the Doctor-Patient relationship is trust. The Ethics of Medicine are not for revision but we fail to distinguish between trash and treasure.

He did not believe in over-relying on tests or statistics. Medicine was complex and needed dual allegiance of the arts and science. The quest for truth was lonely and in the search much trash was sifted and treasure uncovered.

In the practice of therapeutics it was important to know the natural history of the disease and the course it will run without treatment and

[52] Evans, B. Obituary Dr William Evans – Brit. Heart Jr. 1989; 61: 68-70.
[53] Evans, W. 'To tell Trash from Treasure' Wiltshire Memorial Lecture BMA 1961, *Kings College Hospital Gazette*, 1961. Vol. 40 No. 4.

drugs should be submitted to controlled clinical trials with the use of placebos before a drug was routinely prescribed.

'Better to do nothing than something when nothing needs to be done' was often quoted.

'The pages of past history should be burnt into the minds of those who propose to make more, for we should devour first the large store of old knowledge before setting out to discover the new. A worried, hurried, and tired physician is ill equipped to infuse hope and vigour into a dejected patient. A large panel of patients, large attendances at surgeries or outpatient department, a large complement of hospital beds place unjust burdens on the the physician which is inimical to the practice of good medicine'.

Chapter 6

# Visit to a Prime Minister in 1936

After Thomas Lewis decided that he had completed his research on electrocardiography, William Evans decided to pursue the subject as he felt there was more to be gained by study of the topic. Because of his interest, knowledge and research he was asked by Lord Dawson of Penn to visit an important person to give an opinion on his heart under conditions of strictest secrecy.

When he arrived he found his patient was the Prime Minister, Mr. Stanley Baldwin.[54] Rumours had been circulating that Baldwin was a sick man and unfit to lead the Country when Edward VIII became King on the death of King George V. Baldwin was tired, there was disunity in his party, war was threatening and he knew of the King's friendship with Mrs. Simpson. Despite this he was the most popular politician in the country and Tom Jones, Secretary to the Cabinet thought he would remain in office until after the Coronation on 12 May, 1937. Dawson persuaded him to take a holiday in Chequers and asked Dr Evans to meet him in his cottage in Penn and to bring his 'contraption' with him.

Dawson at this time was the Royal Physician, his brother was Editor of the *Times* and both supported the King. Dawson took WE and his Technician to Chequers where after examining the PM an ECG was taken. Dawson regarded Evans as one of his bright young men and he had diagnosed Baldwin as having a heart condition. A communication in the *Times* had indicated that the P.M. might have to resign his Office because of this.

A record was developed and fixed in a boxroom under the stairs, and the ECG showed a deep Q wave and an inverted T wave in lead III. Dr Evans opinion was that it was normal and that Baldwin's heart was healthy and told Baldwin that he intended to use his ECG as that of a healthy heart on the front of his next book. As they returned to

[54] Evans, W. Health as a Political Expediency – *Welsh Medical Gazette*, April 1975 p. 2-5.

Baldwin he asked Dawson who was to give the result, 'You do', he answered.

Was he to reassure him? 'You speak as you find him'.

WE told Baldwin his heart was healthy. Baldwin was delighted[55] and said 'I knew there was nothing wrong with my ticker', and he would be too if things settled down abroad (which Evans understood) and at home (which at the time he did not).

Dawson prescribed a three month holiday which Baldwin[56] spent in Gregynog Hall, Montgomeryshire. Later in the year Baldwin discussed Mrs. Simpson with the King who abdicated on 11 December, 1936.

Baldwin retired after George VI Coronation and was created an Earl and he died in his sleep in 1947 aged 80.

Although Dr Evans name was regularly submitted he never received an Honour. He had shown courage and impartiality of judgement in pronouncing Baldwin's heart healthy and in certain quarters this was never forgiven. Despite making the correct decision, from this time he was excluded from medicine's inner circle.[57]

It was Baldwin's tracing which instigated his investigation into the effect of the height of the diaphragm on the pattern of the ECG in Lead III. The findings were published and led to lead III being included in routine clinical ECG investigation.

[55] David, T. 'Hearts but no Coronets' Plane 72 Dec/Jan 88/89.
[56] Ellis, E. L., 'T.J. A Life of Dr. Thomas Jones, CH'. Gwasg Prifysgol Cymru.
[57] Obituary, Williams Evans, *The Daily Telegraph*, 27 Sept. 1988, p. 25.

Chapter 7

# The Australian Connection and BHF

In 1948 WE had carried out a Lecture Tour in Australia. He had been consulted on plans to accommodate a new Cardiac Investigation Department in the Hallström Institute of Cardiology at the Prince Alfred Hospital, Melbourne, when he visited that department thus establishing a link between the Hallström and the Cardiac Department, London Hospital. The Institute was formally opened on the 22 November 1949.

This was Australia's oldest hospital which had opened at the end of the 18th Century and had always been involved with the management and treatment of heart disease. Physicians with a special interest in cardiology became Honorary Medical Officers of the Hospital. Willie had shown great kindness to all who came from Australia for postgraduate training in the UK. He would welcome them all and give them warm and generous hospitality at his home.

During his visit to Adelaide his wife had seen a tailor to ask if he could make a suit for her husband and had told him 'He's rather portly!' The tailor agreed to the commission and when his wife returned with WE, had told her 'Oh, he is obese'![58]

In 1951[59] there was a move to form the Australian Cardiac Society and the inaugural meeting took place on 27 May 1952 at the Royal Adelaide Hospital. This Society became affiliated to the International Society of Cardiology and had a constitution similar to that of the British Cardiac Society. Six Cardiologists from overseas were invited to become Honorary Foundation members and all accepted. They included Dr W. Evans, Sir John Parkinson, Drs. Charles Lambry, Sam A. Levine, Paul D. White and Paul Wood. The Society changed its name in 1957 to become the Cardiac Society of Australia and New

[58] Evans, W. Personal papers.
[59] Hickie, J. B. & Hickie, K. P. 'Cardiology in Australia & New Zealand' 1990 publ. Cardiac Society of Australia & N.Z.

Zealand. In 1954 William Evans attended the World Congress in Washington D.C. as deputy representative on behalf of the Society.

The Society had the support of Drs. W. Evans and Paul Wood and other distinguished visitors in the formation of the National Heart Foundation of Australia and Dr Evans maintained close links with it. In September 1990, although he had died two years earlier he was sent a copy of a book detailing the historical record of Cardiology in Australia and New Zealand by Hickie & Hickie with the inscription 'We value greatly your contributions over the years to Cardiology and to the Society and hope you will enjoy reading this volume'. Although he was not available to read it I was grateful to read about his valuable contribution.

*British Heart Foundation*

In 1985 Tregaron[60] had a fund raising effort on behalf of the British Heart Appeal and in thanking people for their effort Dr Evans said it showed clearly their interest in the heart and their care of it and as such he counted them individually as his staunch friends.

During a lecture tour of Australia in 1948 he had discovered that there were plans to collect monies to help Doctors combat heart disease. Arrangements were made to knock at every door in the country on a particular Sunday morning in the year to collect money to aid those with heart disease. That knock brought in two million pounds.

'On my return to this country, I sought at the Heart Hospital in London to recruit the Captains of Industry to organise an Appeal to bring in money for research into heart disease in this country and we got half a million pounds. Since then we have continued to increase this so that this year we have collected £10 million. 'What you have done at Tregaron has helped to build up that sum' he told them.

The idea for a British Heart Foundation had come to him in the aeroplane on his return flight from Australia in 1948 but at first he had difficulty in getting it off the ground[61] and had asked Lord Horace Evans who had Palace connections as Physician to Her Majesty Queen Elizabeth II if he would help. 'Leave it to me' he was told.

A Study of 'The History of the British Heart Foundation 1961-1988'[62] reveals that many people and several organisations combined

[60] Tregaron Heart Appeal – Personal papers.
[61] Evans, F. Personal communication.
[62] Matthews, D. N. 'Fighting Heart Disease'. 'The History of the British Heart Foundation' 1961-1988, Blackwell, 1990.

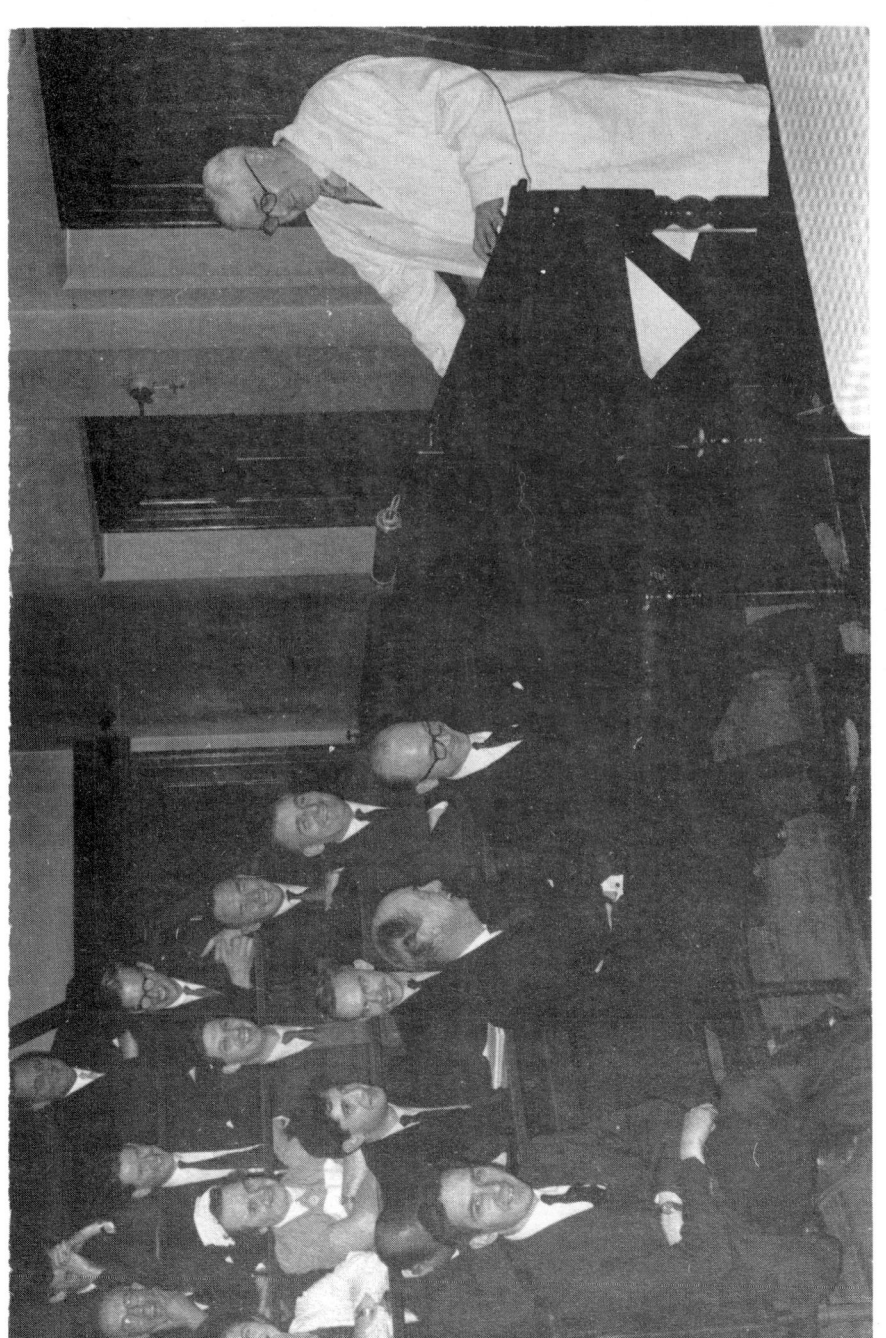

Humour in the Lecture Theatre.

*(Photograph by permission of Miss Frances Evans.)*

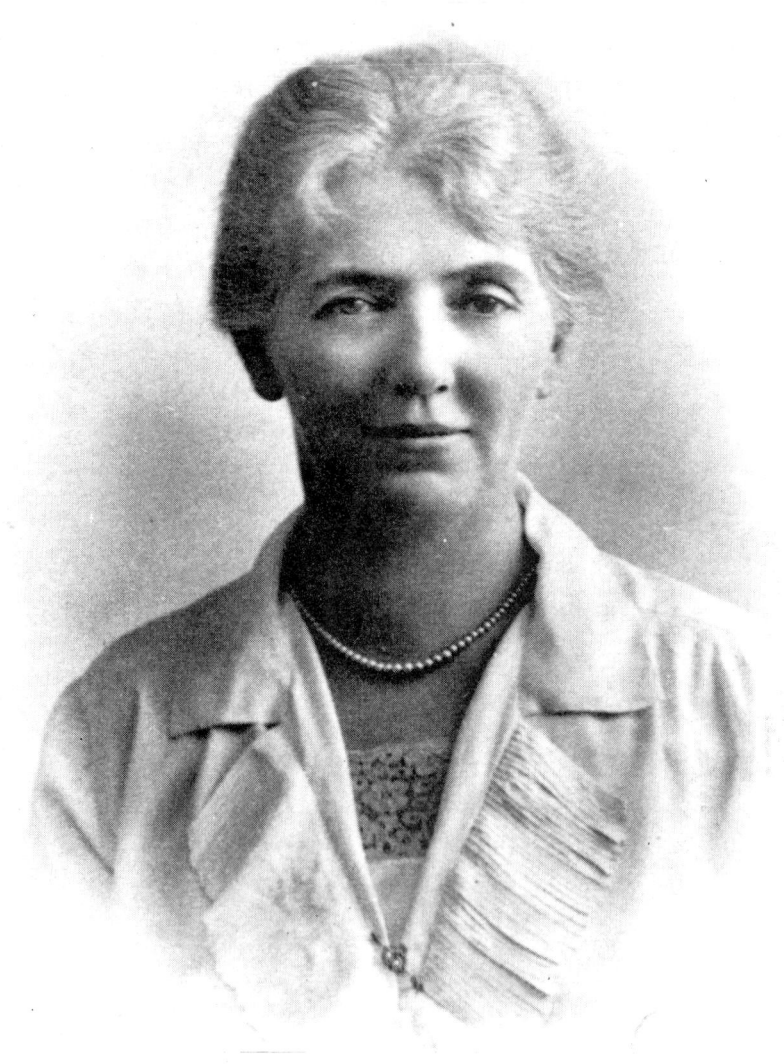

Christina Evans – his wife.
*(Photograph by permission of Miss Frances Evans.)*

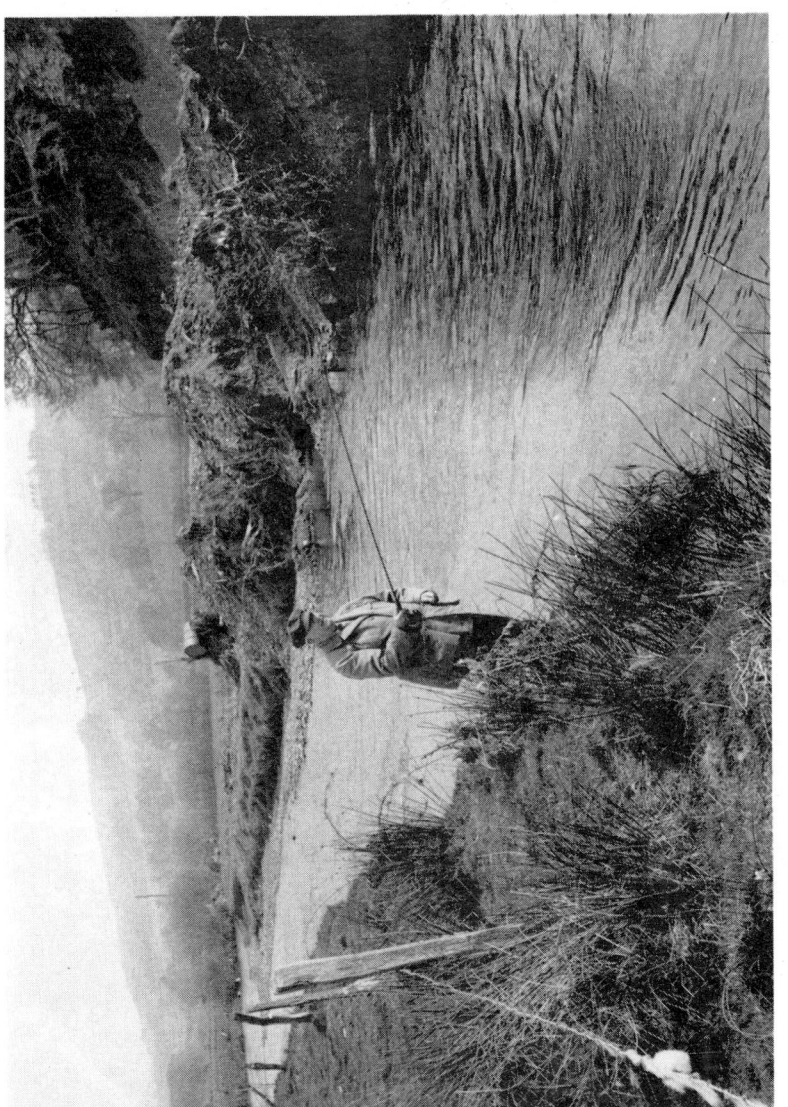

Fishing in the Teifi.

*(Photograph by permission of Miss Frances Evans.)*

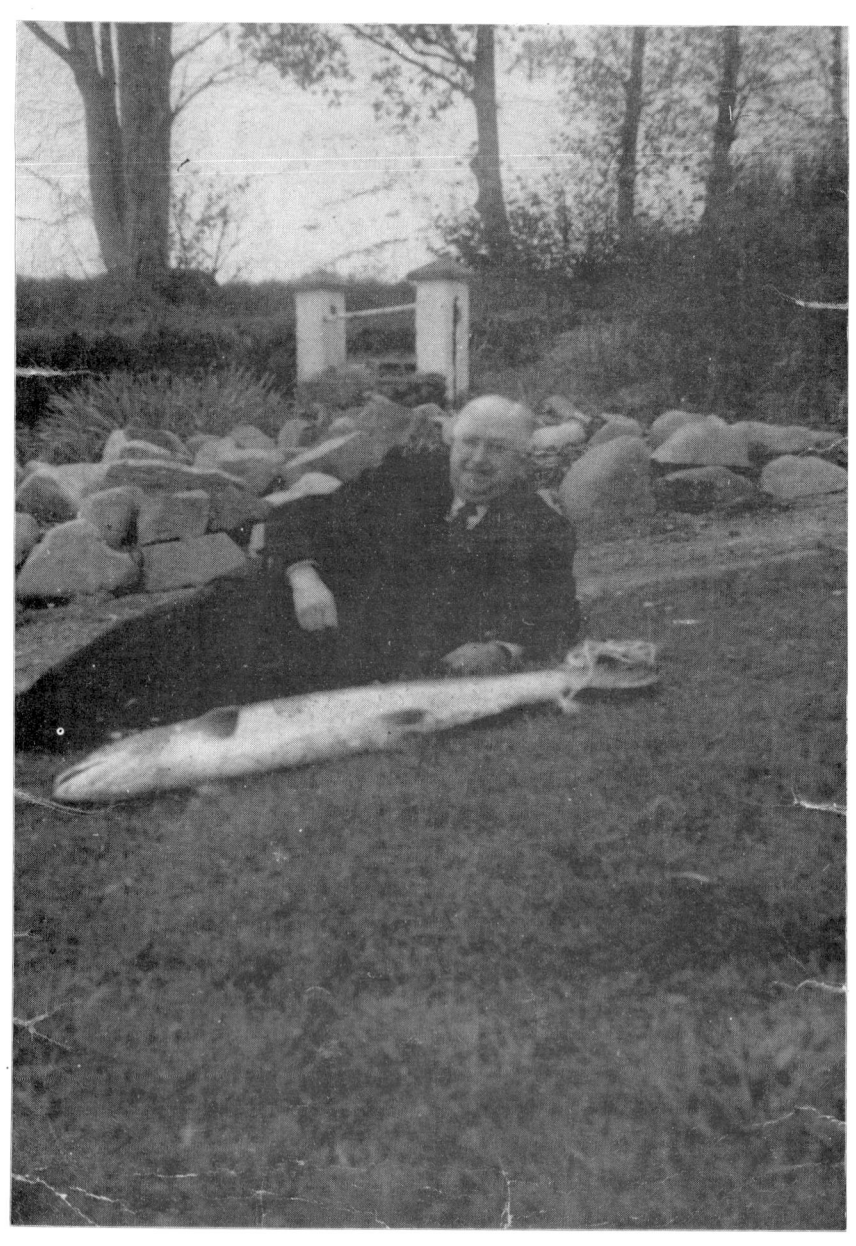

The Trophy.
*(Photograph by permission of Miss Frances Evans.)*

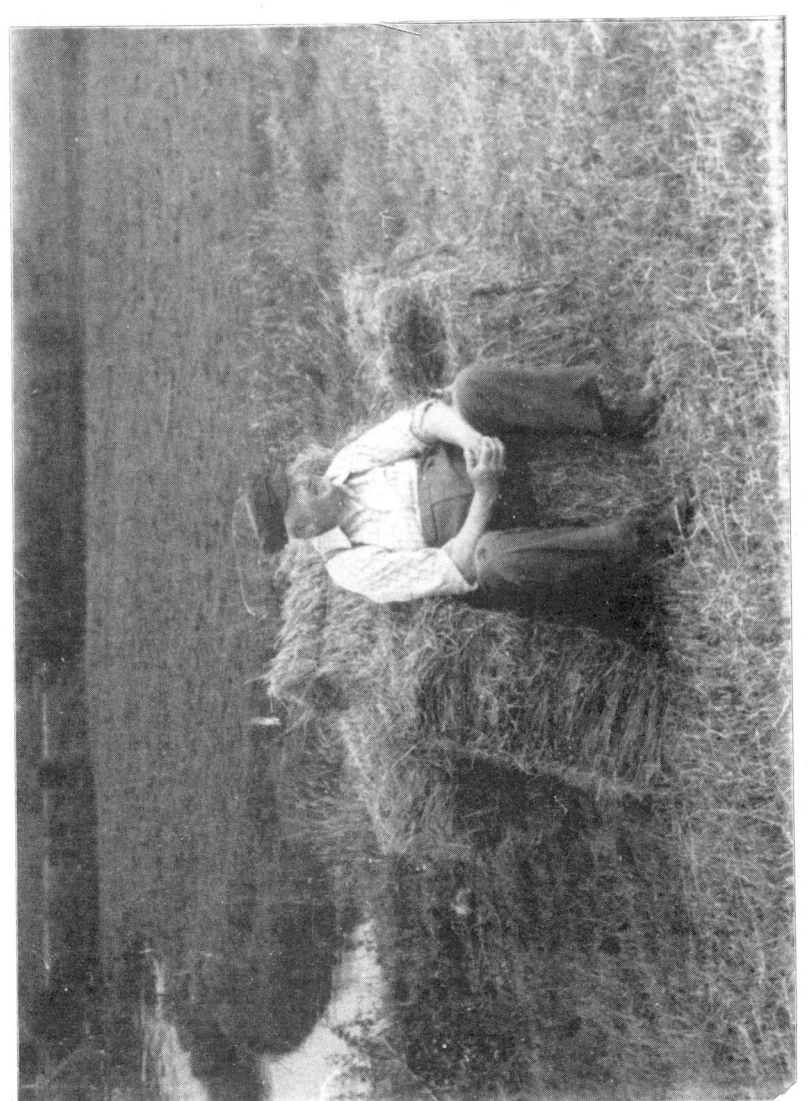

Harvesting – Back Home.

*(Photograph by permission of Miss Frances Evans.)*

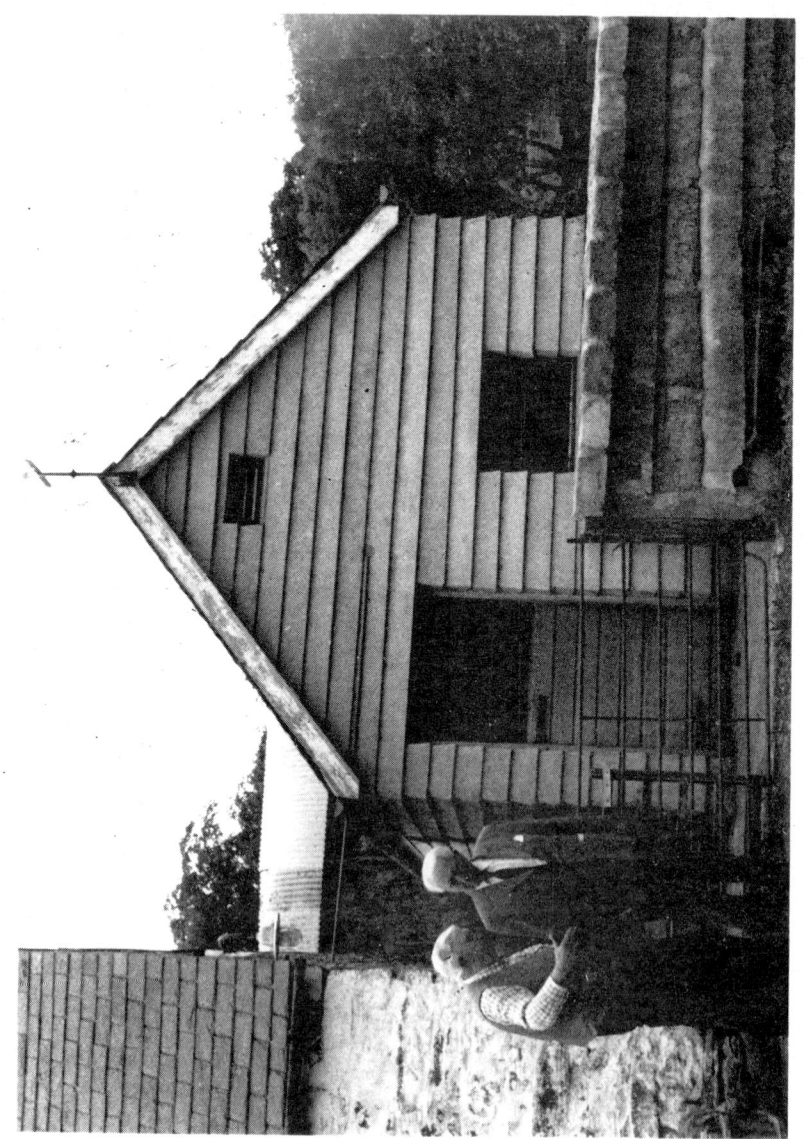

The calf shed he built.

*(Photograph by permission of Miss Frances Evans.)*

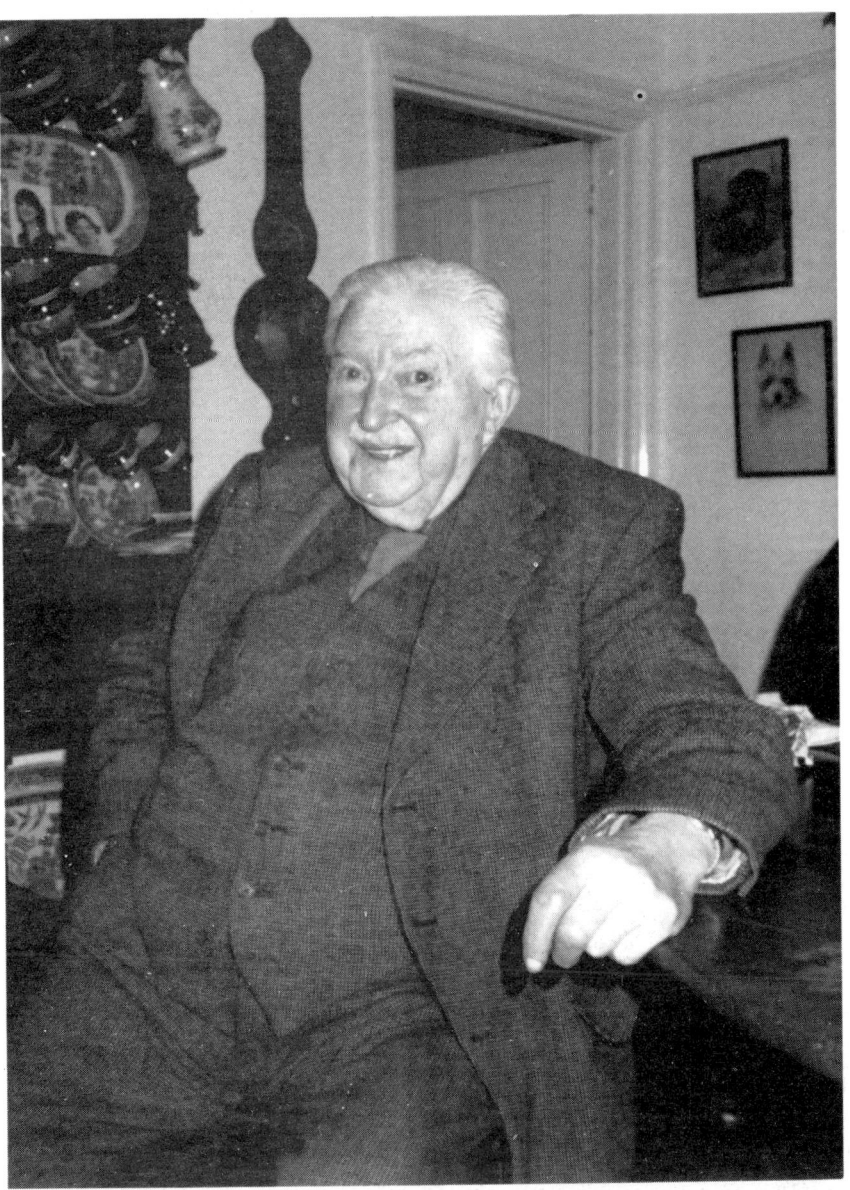

In Old Age.

*(Photograph by permission of Miss Frances Evans.)*

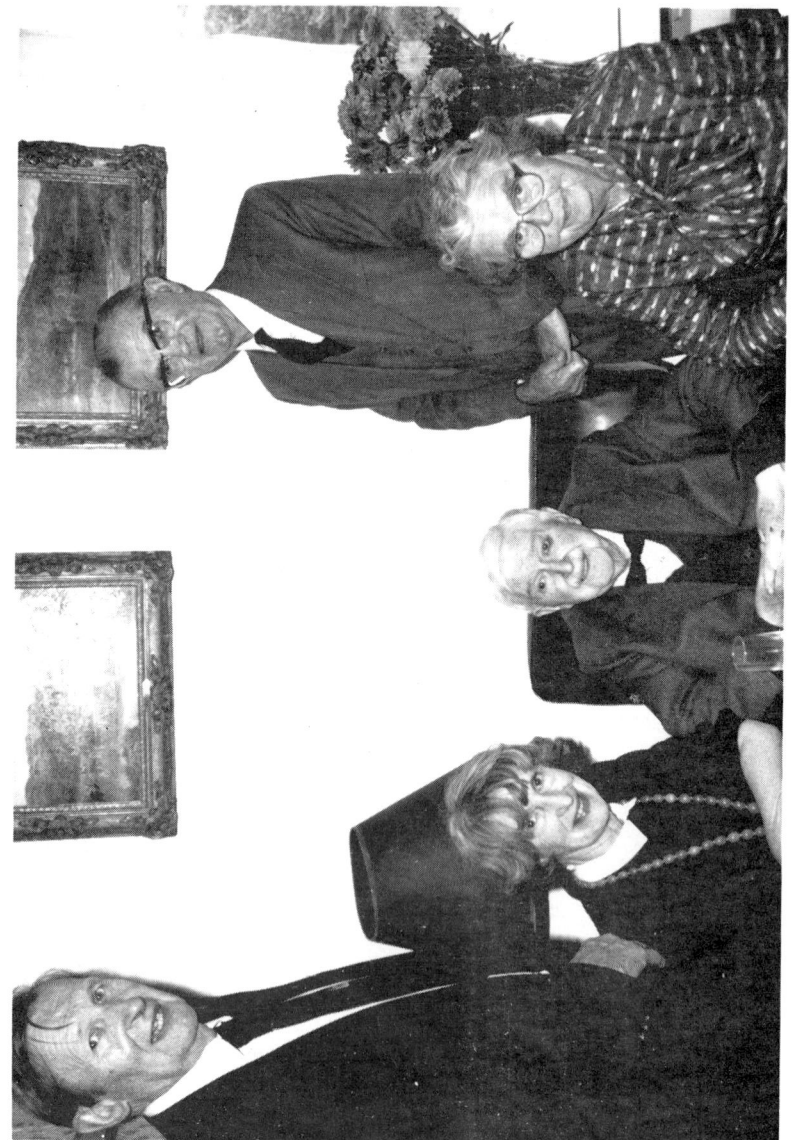

Family Group.

*(Photograph by permission of Miss Frances Evans.)*

to create the BHF from a common desire to provide funds for research into heart disease. The two organisations which played major roles were the British Cardiac Society and the Chest and Heart Foundation supported by the Royal Colleges and Medical Research Council.

The British Cardiac Society formed in 1937 had grown from the Cardiac Club of Great Britain which was formed in 1922 with 15 members and Sir Thomas Lewis as its first Chairman. It had changed its name to the Cardiac Society of Great Britain and Ireland and then to the British Cardiac Society with sixty ordinary members and twenty-five associate members with the object of advancement of knowledge of disease of the heart and circulation for the benefit of the public. WE was one of the Founder Members who was a member of Council twice in 1942-46 and 1956-1960, Chairman in 1965 and had been elected an Honorary Member in 1962.

The Chest and Heart Association is a charity which developed from the National Association for the Prevention of Tuberculosis which had been in existence for sixty years before changing its name in 1959. In 1975 it added Stroke to its title becoming the Chest, Heart and Stroke Association. When it became the Chest and Heart Association it had plans to launch an appeal for one million pounds to finance heart research. At the same time the British Cardiac Society was exploring the possibility of creating a fund raising body and the President, Dr Maurice Campbell, had raised two possibilities, either that the Society should form an association to raise money for research or they should seek co-operation with the National Association for the Prevention of Tuberculosis.

The Council decided to appoint a committee to determine what steps should be taken to form a new association for raising money for research and had informal discussions with the President of the Royal College of Physicians and Secretary of the Medical Research Council. They recommended that such an organisation be established and should consist of medical and lay members and that the number of lay members should not exceed the number of medical members. A Council meeting of the British Cardiac Society decided to promote the creation of a British Heart Foundation which would become a separate entity but in the meantime they fostered it through a Founding Committee of four of their Council members.

It was Dr Evans who proposed at a meeting of the Council of the British Cardiac Society in the Spring of 1957 under the item 'any other business' that a National Heart Foundation be formed. A short discussion took place and the Secretary, Dr Patrick Mouncey was requested to place it on the agenda of the next meeting. At the next meeting a Founding Committee was formed of Dr Maurice Campbell, Dr Evan Bedford, Dr Paul Wood and Dr William Evans. At this stage it became necessary to win the support of the Chest and Heart Association with Dr Harley Williams, its Secretary, a tough negotiator. It was arranged that Drs. Evans and Paul Wood would meet Dr Harley Williams and at the meeting Harley Williams agreed to drop their appeal and also agreed that an appeal be launched for the British Heart Foundation as an independent body. The Foundation was fortunate to have in Dr Evans an illustrious and enthusiastic pioneer in its formative years and his support throughout his professional life and retirement while his health lasted. He responded generously to requests to address medical and social fund-raising events.

On receiving a letter from Professor Shillingford in 1984 telling him that the Foundation's annual income had exceeded £6 million he wrote back saying 'to have been in the van of a movement which collects from the general public a sum of money exceeding £6 million in a single year in support of a crusade which aims to deal with ailing hearts, creates a belief that the Nation's heart continues to beat unerringly true'.[63]

The first meeting of the Founding Committee was held at the Royal College of Physicians on 8th September 1959. It was agreed that Dr William Evans and Dr Paul Wood should serve on a sub-committee to continue negotiations with the Chest and Heart Association and the Chairman and Secretary agreed to act as a sub-committee to initiate the necessary legal steps to establish the BHF.

At the fourth meeting of the Founding Committee held at BMA House on the 18th January 1960, when the composition of Council was the main item for discussion, Dr Harley Williams suggested that a 5000 word statement of intent and objectives, couched in lay terms was needed for publicity in advance of the appeal and Drs William Evans and Paul Wood were entrusted with the task. The resulting printed leaflet was entitled 'The Heart Problem' which was the first publication produced by the Foundation.

At the fifth meeting of the Founding Committee on 2 May 1960 an Appeal Policy Committee of six was set up which included William and he with Lord Evans became Vice-Chairmen. This met on six

---

[63] Evans, W. Letter to Prof. Shillingford – Personal papers.

occasions and was dissolved on 31st January 1961. The sixth and final meeting of the Founding Committee was held on the 6th February 1961, the next meeting being the first meeting of the Council of the BHF. An Executive Committee was appointed consisting of members of the Appeal Policy Committee which included Dr WE.

The Foundation became a reality on 28th July 1961 when the Board of Trade issued a Certificate of Incorporation as a Company.

Lord Horace Evans approached leading Industrialists and business men to enlist their support for the Foundation and organised a Dinner Party at his home on 17th July 1961 which was an important milestone. (Appendix VII) A second meeting at Lord Evans' home on 5 February 1962 resulted in the formation of a powerful appeal committee with Lord Evans and Dr W. Evans as Vice-Chairmen.

In 1980 the BHF had given £300,000 to endow the Sir Thomas Lewis Chair of Cardiology in Cardiff with Professor Andrew Henderson appointed. The cheque was handed to the University at an inaugural meeting on 24 November and WE had attended the ceremony having been taken to Cardiff by car by Dr Rhys. WE attended the twenty fifth Anniversary Dinner of the BHF at the Cavalry and Guards Club despite ill-health on 17 July 1986 and was seated between Sir Cyril Clarke and Professor Jack Shillingford. He was the only one of two still alive who were at the original dinner twenty-five years earlier. When he died in 1988 he was the last of the four original members of the Founding Committee to do so.

# Chapter 8

# Way of Life

Byron Evans summed WE up, in a letter to the *Western Mail*[64] which had asked for names of Welsh Greats, succinctly as :–

> A humble Welsh speaking Welshman of International fame who until 1960 was the greatest teacher of Cardiology in the World. He had been invited to give lectures of distinction in the Commonwealth, Europe and the USA. He was the author of five standard books on Cardiology and over 100 papers. He had written the Diary of a Welsh Swagman which gained the approbation of the Australian Education Authority as part of the curriculum on Australian History. He had held office as High Sheriff of Cardiganshire, was an Honourary Druid and had received the Honorary Fellowship of the Royal Society of Medicine.

Always interested in research and among his references to it is:

> Man is being preferred to the rat for investigation for two reasons, he is a more docile animal and has better veins.

also

> Through the years I have been amazed at the healing properties of coloured water, especially the red kind.

As David Mendel[65] wrote

> It is virtuoso performance, humanity and wit which make men into giants. It is not the projected image but the polished skills as performers which make men first rate.

---

[64] Evans, B. Correspondence, *Western Mail*. 9 Nov. 1981.
[65] Mendel, D. Personal Correspondence.

Reflecting philosophically WE wrote

There is no loss so finite as lost opportunity, the search for it is futile.

One's past is either a dustbin of lost opportunities or the granary of accumulated wisdom.

Immortality depends largely on other people's memories.

From reading his papers I found out unexpected facets of his life. He was a Governor of the Gillete London Marathon in 1982 and in the programme listed as Chairman of the British Amateur Athletic Board.[66]

In 1977 in the Dean's Report[67] in the London Hospital Gazette, the Dean had pointed out that 'in this year's sports Willie Evans easily won the Consultant's Race. In fairness to his successors it must be stated that a combination of handicap, a good get-away, gathering momentum and less than excellent hearing resulted in his failing to heed the recall for a false start occasioned by Mike Floyer's still youthful eagerness. The sight of Willie breasting the tape alone was an inspiration to the young and a relief to at least one of his old students who had visions of bending over a prostrate body repeating to himself as taught long ago – Can I hear the first heart sound?'

He was an advocate for exercise and advised a Conference for Executives in 1964[68] to sell the car, buy a dog, walk, or garden. 'Do not worry, walk'. There is a new disease of disuse he told them. We have lost our self reliance and do not acknowledge the healing powers of nature. Pill taking has made us slaves of fashion; a placebo and reassurance is often excellent. He quotes from John Dryden's advice in 1680:–

'Better to hunt in fields, for health unbought, than the doctor for a nauseous draught'. We do not acknowledge the healing powers of nature which are powerful.

One article in the *Observer Magazine*[69] on 4 June 1967 which was devoted to 'your heart and its future' was by a Cardiologist in Harley Street known as 'the grand old man of Cardiology' but not named. The sentiments expressed were those of WE though why he should remain

---

[66] The Gillette London Marathon Official Programme, 9 May 1982, p. 3.
[67] Dean's Report *London Hospital Gazette* 1977 No. 2 p. 17.
[68] Conference for Executives 1964. 'Sell Car and Walk' – Leader, Times – 17.4.64.
[69] 'Your Heart and its Future', *Observer Magazine* – 4th June 1967, p. 29.

anonymous when he had expressed the views in print elsewhere I am not sure. He maintained that the coronary arteries were inaccessible to the surgeon and likely to remain so, and the management and treatment of those with diseased arteries was the responsibility of the Cardiologist. Reassurance should take pride of place. The patient should be encouraged to resume habits of work and hobbies. A change of occupation should be discouraged. Exercise is encouraged with the aid of glyceryl trinitrate. Excess weight should be lost but he had not seen proof that animal fats and sugar caused coronary arterial disease. Undue regard to statistics should be discouraged. He did not think smoking caused coronary disease but it was an unsavoury habit! He believed in 'A little of what you fancy does you good'. He did not like the advice 'you should lead a normal life but do not go out alone, that is not normal'. 'Too many do nots – the cure is in the head'. 'We should have equanimity for life and not worry about our weight'.

He also wrote an article on Safe Foods which was published in the *Farmers Weekly* after his retirement as 'Hearty eaters can take heart'[70] expressing similar sentiments.

He regarded statistics as 'that unreliable tool in the hands of the epidemiologist which can build out of a hillock of probability, a mountain of presumption and conjecture'.

He regarded as misguided and foolish and patently mischievous Committees attempting to influence Government to decree that polyunsaturated fats should replace animal fats to prevent coronary disease. Governments should not interfere with staple diets especially of children, but he gave the advice 'Arise from the table feeling you could eat more'.

Longevity depends on the state of coronary, cerebral and renal arteries. Atheroma starts early. His family had lived to old age and The Trefecel Diaries (1846-1947) show their diet was healthy. An American asked WE, 'Aren't you worried about cholesterol?' 'Of course I am' came the reply, 'I can't get enough of it'! Of course he was not always right!

Many speeches gave his philosophy on life. In 1961 at Llandaff Cathedral in an address to the Rose League[71] he quoted Sir Ernest Morris, House Governor of London Hospital.

---

[70] Evans, W. 'Hearty eaters can take heart' *Farmers Weekly*, March 3, 1978, p. 102.
[71] Evans, W. 'Bowl of Roses' – Llandaff Cathedral 30.4.61. Personal papers.

'All manner of medicines had been tried and had failed but a bowl of roses got him better'. Learn to care for one another, to live for one another as well as with one another. Chivalry is spontaneous selfless devotion to succour the troubled. Patients need to be lifted from despondent loneliness.

The needs of today are those of the frail, who should be at home not in a Home; and neglected youth caused by disruption of the serenity of the home by the mother out working.

He invites his audience to form a Rose League to bridge the gap between the old and young. This is to practice wayside religion, encouraging children to run errands and promoting the idea of street wardens.

In 1962 he gave an address on Discipline and Discipleship at St. Martins in the Field on behalf of the Chest and Heart Association.

In a speech to Tregaron YFC whose crest showed a man following a plough he took his title 'Ploughing a Straight Furrow'.[72] The plough has been used as a symbol of great goodness or 'of good intent'. For him it meant following the call for discipline and discipleship – rare commodities in present Society. A disciple can not be one unless he has discipline – both words now out of fashion. In the home and school they are the cornerstone of character. 'Spare the rod and spoil the child'. Punishment should be corrective and he was in favour of corporal punishment. We need to imbue the young with the value of work which is health giving spice of life. As Pope said 'want of occupation is not rest, a mind at leisure is a mind distressed'.

Liberty and freedom are not synonymous – Liberty is a disciplined freedom and one needed discipline in one's moral relationships. A passport for life is to run a straight furrow with assiduity, application, aspiration in work, honesty, selflessness, compassion and chastity.

He gave three attestations: cultivate gentleness in your dealings, stand guard over your character, shepherd your reputation.

WE kept a red hardbacked book of Maxims: Axioms, Quotations which had an Index of eleven pages catalogued alphabetically followed by 135 pages of sayings in neat, meticulous writing. Many quotations are from the Bible, Shakespeare and other Literary figures including Cicero and Hippocrates. They are pithy, pertinent and sometimes impertinent with the clear intent to debunk pomposity and humbug.

---

[72] Evans, W. 'Ploughing a Straight Furrow' – Talk to YFC Tregaron and District.

No. 114 reads 'School masters have been known to report that a boy has a kind disposition, but not clever, and so could make a good doctor'.

WE notes 'it is what we need today, kind not clever doctors'.

No. 159 'An after dinner speech helps people in different ways. Some rise from it greatly stimulated others wake from it greatly refreshed'.

Work, death and achievement have the greatest number of quotes. In Cardigan County Eisteddfod YFC at Tregaron[73] in 1973 he talked about the changes he found back home after half a century away. He does not like the term Dyfed – 'do not allow Sir Aberteifi, Ceredigion and the Cardi to be submerged' he told them. He does not like change in customs and practice on the farm – mechanisation, afforestation, pesticides, fertilisers instead of organic farming, dehorning which was un-natural and cruel, pollution of rivers, extraction of water, pollution in farm buildings. He makes a plea to preserve farming as a way of life not just as a business as we should regard the humanitarian as well as utilitarian aspects. 'Have regard for the aesthetic and do not get too specialised'.

In his Presidential Address to the Science Club[74] of Tregaron County School in January 1970 he told them 'whatever position or post you take up in life you must not make it hum-drum, and your continued quest for truth will always bring you the prize of rare happiness'. 'The quest for truth can be a most exciting and romantic experience. The born investigator is a born enthusiast'. 'Research is to search again, so that an accepted truth may be shown to be untrue. The combination of chance and vision in the quest of truth goes to form the syndrome of serendipity'.

He quotes Robert Watson-Watt, a relative of James Watt, noticing a disturbance on his cathode ray tube glanced out of the window and saw an aircraft flying overhead. He set out with added zeal to perfect radar (radiodetecting and ranging) by this chance observation which years later was used in the war to bring down enemy bombers.

When he opened the new St. John Ambulance and Red Cross Headquarters in Aberystwyth in 1964,[75] which had been converted

[73] Evans, W. Cardiganshire County Eisteddfod, Tregaron 1973.
[74] Evans, W. 'Chance & Vision in Research' Science Club Tregaron County School 1970, 13 January. Personal papers.
[75] Evans, W. Opening of St. John and Red Cross headquarters, *Welsh Gazette*, October 1, 1964.

from a chapel, he said that admiration for the beautiful was giving way to hideous, vulgar and satanic conditions produced by increased affluence, automation and ignorance of how to use leisure, along with neglect of Religious Education. He would ask University College of Wales Aberystwyth to found a Chair of Leisure to help people cope with added free time.

WE's opinions were strongly held and forcefully expressed. He was heard with respect even if people did not always agree with him but his underlying motive was the abiding concern of a wise and kindly physician. He never let his medical students forget the need to support and sustain the sufferer.

He thought pre-speaking apprehension was not a bad thing because it indicated an anxiety lest the material which the speaker has assembled has not sufficient merit to lay before a gathering which has paid him or her the compliment of coming to listen. Churchill, MacMillan and Lord Dawson of Penn had it and Shakespeare described it

'I've tremor cardis, my heart dances,
but not for joy'

His wife had predeceased him in 1964 and he had written 'An understanding wife in the security of a happy home is the doctor's greatest ally and more precious than any well trained almoner in a highly organised rehabilitation centre'.

He had married Christina Downie, 30.12.84 – 17.10.64, of the Downie Crab Apple family at All Souls, Langham Place on 10 February 1936. Christina Downie was born in Liverpool. Her father John Downie was an engineer and as a hobby was interested in Crab Apples and one is named after him – The Downie Crab Apple – which is good for Crab Apple Jelly and there is a specimen in the garden at Tyndomen.

Christina had been a Nurse, Sister and Tutor at the London Hospital from 1914-1935 and after her death WE made a general bequest to the Hospital League of Nurses. The money was invested and the interest used annually to purchase books for the Nurses Library as during her lifetime Christina had sent an annual gift to the Library.

She and WE were interested in gardening and in the mid 30's they bought a farm near Eastbourne letting the land but keeping the house and garden, selling eventually in 1955. He described his home as a fastness giving a sense of security during his childhood and in his marriage and in Tregaron he had Frances to look after him. When he was working he would return at the end of each day to a home of unruffled serenity and calm 'over which presides a rare companion' – Chris. She would do handwork or reading while he wrote and would offer a suitable word if he was stuck.

They also had big apartments in London. 19 Cavendish Square 1935-1956 and later one in St. John's Wood; in 1956 he took over the tenancy of 69 Northgate.

It was a happy marriage but on 15 October 1964 – General Election Day – she had collapsed and became unconscious in the Polling Booth. She was taken to St. John and St. Elizabeth Hospital where she died on 17 October at 2 a.m. aged 80. Her funeral was held on 21 October at Marylebone Crematorium. They had been married 28 years and had no children.

In his writings he showed how he had coped with loneliness and loss of companionship which followed.

Chapter 9

# Retirement

On 24 November 1967 he retired from Medical Practice, his chattels were loaded for Wales on 4 December and unloaded at Bryndomen on the 6th December.

He was home and soon in the swing of speaking to local societies of W.I., N.F.U., Liberal Association, Inner Wheel, Round Table, Cymdeithas Cenhadol, Y.F.C., Mother's Union, British Legion, Soroptomists and Medical Women's Federation. He was also invited to give Medical Lectures and was sought as an After-Dinner Speaker. He was invited to become President or Vice-President of Local Societies and responded generously when asked for his assistance. He also entertained his many friends and colleagues who called to see him.

He was High Sheriff of Cardiganshire 1959-60 and used both Luncheon occasions as a platform for his views which were reported in the Press. At his first luncheon on the 18 June 1959 at St. David's College, Lampeter, Reverend George Noakes was his Chaplain. George Noakes was Vicar of Tregaron at the time and later became Bishop of St. David's and Archbishop of Wales. WE spoke of Welsh Nationhood; that the Nation was great and must remain so by exercising discipline, cherishing the language and integrity. Freedom and Liberty were won through selflessness. He was afraid that there was moral laxity in Society,[76] that morality should start at home where parents should guard it. Good manners were important and he had spoken at Tregaron County School in December 1959 on the Ten Commandments of Good Manners.

He had a busy year. On 9 October 1959 he had declared the Election Result with Roderic Bowen getting back as M.P. for Cardiganshire and on 3 October had spoken at the Tuberculosis Eisteddfod in Aberystwyth – The Silent Eisteddfod: which was for Arts and Crafts.

---

[76] Evans, W. High Sheriff hits out at Moral Laxity, *Cambrian News*, 4 March 1960.

On 4 August 1960 he had been installed as an Honorary Member of the Gorsedd of Bards taking the name Amnon III. This was reported in *The Times* on the 5 August along with the fact that the Gorsedd had been driven indoors by rain and there was no Chairing.

In September he had chaired a Panel on Coronary Heart Disease at the European Congress of Cardiology in Rome.

He retired from the National Heart Hospital on 24 November 1960 and from the London Hospital on 31 December. On the subject of retirement he said 'Retirement marks the end of gainful employment but it is the port of entry into a period of rewarding enjoyment; an emergence from the competitive race with its hazards and its hurdles into the calm fields which provide for contemplative soliloquy'.

He had returned to his roots and to the life he had enjoyed during his childhood.

He kept a diary from 1969-1973;[77] a five year diary in red leather hard backed 4″ x 6″ book form which had a clasp which could be locked by a key, and inside the inscription read 'This diary belongs to William Evans, Bryndomen, Tregaron'. Each page was divided into five horizontal areas for the same date but different consecutive years. In it the weather was chronicled daily and also his forecast for the following day which was not always correct.

In this diary I discovered his masonry skills in building the calf shed and pens at Tyndomen, the dog kennels, concrete paths in the garden, building the pillar for the plaque in the meadow and tiling the bathroom.

He enjoyed his garden and cutting thistles in the fields. His gardening year started at the beginning of March by planting shallots and giving the roses bone meal. Later in the month he planted potatoes, gooseberry, peach and plum and in April sowed lettuce, spring onions, leeks, beet, swedes, onion, parsnip, thyme, parsley, aubrietia and anemone. He drew a picture of his vegetable plot and noted when the lawn was first cut and when the hedge was layered.

He notes the arrival and departure of the swallows and when he heard the cuckoo. He was interested in the farm stock, the treatment of footrot in sheep, when lambs were bought and sold; brucellosis testing of the Welsh Black Cattle and dosing for fluke and worm and the application against warble fly. The dates of harrowing and threshing were included in the yearly cycle of farm life.

[77] Evans, W. Five Year Diary – Personal papers.

He was domesticated and did not have help in the house. He could cook and entertain his friends and one entry confirmed that he had given Byron Evans cold ham and chips for supper followed by blackberry tart. He made curtains and hung them after he had painted a bedroom and laid the carpet. He chopped sticks for the fire and he mended the incinerator.

He was a keen fisherman interested in Teifi Brown Trout and was a member of the South West Wales Angling Association. As an astute fisherman he said 'It is not the type of fly that is important but the way it is presented to the fish'.

His working days were long and full and in the evenings he would write out the work for the morrow and say 'Plan today, plod tomorrow'. After a day's physical work he would continue to write.

He did not own a car, did not drive and relied on public transport or the kindness of friends to get around. To get to Wrexham on 20 February 1970 he had taken a bus from Tregaron to Aberystwyth then the train to Shrewsbury where he had been met by his friend Dr Kiloh and had spent the night at his home. He had lectured in Wrexham on the 20th and had commented in his diary of the difficulty in getting the car out of the hotel yard because of ice and snow. He returned to Aberystwyth on the 21st where he was guest speaker at the British Legion Dinner and the following day gave the BMA Lecture on 'Abiding Truths in the diagnosis and treatment of Heart Disease'. This was a trip away from home where he combined three talks with staying with friends – enjoyment and good time management.

He was generous in speaking to many medical and lay societies. He was Guest Speaker at the Medical Womens Federation Council Dinner in Swansea in 1973 when Miss Catrin Williams FRCS was President. She was the first Welsh woman and Consultant ENT Surgeon in North Clwyd to become President of the MWF. He attended a Symposium in London on Naval Medicine and spoke at the Royal College of Physicians on 'HMS Ganges Scheme'.

He was equally prepared to talk to local Women's Institutes, Merched y Wawr, Young Farmers Clubs, Cymru'r Groes, Rotarians, Cymdeithas Ceredigion, Inner Wheel, Tregaron Book Club as well as giving the Holy Week address at St. Caron's Church. The topics covered ranged from 'Discipline & Discipleship', 'Keeping up with the Joneses', 'Serendipity', 'Chance and Vision in Discovery', 'Loneliness', and 'Authorship'.

As well as 'Journey to Harley Street' he wrote 'Back Home' which

Dr Hugh Herbert took on his behalf to a London Publisher on 13 February 1973 but this was not published. In the preamble to his Autobiography he had said that at best an Autobiography is an exercise in self-indulgence. 'To write a book about someone else requires unbiased judgement, to write about oneself demands impeccable honesty. The reading of an Autobiography never gives as much pleasure as its writing; its composition has been an exciting creation; the reader may class it as drab mediocrity'. He pointed out that the pen had been a necessary adjunct to his life in prose and poem. When he was High Sheriff of Cardiganshire he had been appointed an Honorary Member of the Order of Druids and chose Amnon III as his bardic name as his grandfather had been Amnon II. Although I had read that he had published a book of poems this was untrue although some had been published in his Autobiography, some in Cerddi Cerngoch and some in newspapers. In 1970 Frances received a Prince of Wales award for 'Cornel y Domen' and he went with her to Llandudno to witness her receiving the plaque from Prince Charles. In January 1971 he and Frances visited the meadow and decided where a pillar was to be erected at 'Cornel y Domen' to commemorate the award. This is opposite Bryndomen at the head of the lane. WE met Prince Charles twice, first at a luncheon in Llandrindod Wells and then at the Royal Welsh Show but he does not go into any details about this in the diary.

He was a Liberal who regularly attended the Annual Association Dinner in Lampeter and the Welsh Liberal Conference. He was presiding officer at Lampeter, when High Sheriff, when Roderic Bowen, Q.C., a personal friend, was returned as member of Parliament for Cardiganshire. It was Roderic Bowen who proposed his Health at the Dinners held to celebrate his 80 and 90 birthdays. He was also a member of the Court of Governors of University College of Wales, Aberystwyth.

Through the diary I read of Dr Arwyn Williams' funeral on 22 June 1973. I started my professional career in 1949 by doing a fortnight's locum for Dr A. Williams as he entrusted me with his General Practice in Tregaron while he took a holiday. I stayed in comfort in his home with a housekeeper to cook my meals, a chauffeur to drive his car, (I could not drive at the time) and luckily no tremendous medical problems arose though I sent one patient with suspected appendicitis into hospital. It was a good start.

In the diary I also learnt of WE's ailments. In 1971 he had Lumbago which got worse after gardening which he wrote 'was a silly thing to do'.

In March 1972 he had cardiac pain which the ECG confirmed was probably a spasm. He was in bed for eleven days and a week after getting up he gave the BMA Lecture in Cardiff to 150 people which he wrote was a great success. On the way there by car he had visited Lloyds Bank Dowlais where he had worked so many years previously. Later in the year he complained of indigestion.

I mentioned earlier that he had a haemorrhage after qualifying and in 1955 he had a Hemicolectomy by Lloyd Davies for a growth in the colon and in 1959 a Laparotomy. He also had a Tonsillectomy as an adult.

When he went into the Middlesex to have a cancer removed they did an ECG on one of the photographic machines in which the line wobbled up and down a slit. David Mendel went to see him and asked how he was, and he said that he had spotted that his T wave in Lead 3 was upside down, so he took a deep breath to stop them fussing about it!

He loved the company of his friends and old students some of whom regularly called to see him as did the General Practitioners in the vicinity. Books and writing were important but a gift of a Television from medical friends was rejected and returned to Radio Rentals. His friends had been concerned about his loneliness but his answer was 'Loneliness as a lone complaint is a preventable illness and its specific antidote is continued occupation'. He maintained that he had better and more constructive things to do.

On 29 November 1975 his assistants entertained him to dinner in Cardiff to celebrate his 80th birthday. Eirian Williams had invited him to a dinner at the Cadena Cafe, Tiger Bay and 'Byron speaks highly of it' and 'The 4th is Max Boyce' he was told. Of course the dinner was at Cardiff Arms Park and he said it was a tremendous thrill for him to see so many of his old students. Octogenarians are in a class apart he said, better endowed and aristocrats of the race, have special genes for survival, are supernormal paragons of Society, patricians of the upper ten physiological elect and biological elite. His secret he said in a radio interview was that as a baby he drank gallons of Cardiganshire's soft water. As an adult he ate animal fat rich in energising esters.

On two occasions he had been regarded as dead. The first reported him missing in France in the First World War and the second in 1970 when David Short of Aberdeen received a letter from abroad regretting his passing.

He believed it was friendship which drew them all together. As defined by a Schoolboy Friendship is shown by someone who knows you but loves you just the same. His greatest reward was making friends and he thanked them for 'their attendance, friendship, loyalty and continued help to uphold and to promote the sanctity and the unassailability of clinical medicine for the abiding benefit of our fellow-man'.

When erecting a stone wall at Tyndomen he became ill and was admitted to Withybush Hospital under Dr Eirian Williams, semi-delirious with $\alpha$-Influenza Virus. He had no food for a week and on the 9th day food was offered but his dentures were missing. Sister rang the Laundry where they were found and returned with a Primula Pseudodenticulata!

In his 80's he had a stroke after repairing a wall and was never the same afterwards, becoming very feeble. At the end he again had rectal bleeding but did not want resuscitation when admitted to Withybush under the care of Dr Eirian Williams and where he died. In a Lecture to the BMA in Swansea[78] in 1965 he had scorned the notion that regular medical examinations could be given to twenty three million Britons over forty as in his estimation he felt it would induce morbid anxiety. The best judge of a man's health was his spouse, secretary or supervisor. 'Our function is to heal the sick, not sicken the healthy'.

He had returned from London to the sort of life he had wished for as a young man and despite the loss of his wife he appears to have had a contented retirement: happy with his lot, cared for by Frances and visited regularly by many friends.

In an interview in the *Cambrian News*[79] in December 1982 when he was 87 he talks of the natural polled Welsh Black herd and Welsh Mountain Ewe Stock. Before going to bed he would write out what he needed to do on the morrow and tick them off as the tasks were done. He would get up at 6 a.m. and potter in Tyndomen if the weather was favourable but if wet he would write. He had a full day everyday and quoted 'Compulsive contemplation and Compulsive occupation' as his philosophy in life.

His life and work was influenced by his religious beliefs and he read a Chapter of the Bible each night before going to sleep.

He was asked by Dr Hilary Loxdale, President of Soroptomists International in Carmarthen to reopen the refurbished Greenhill flats for the elderly. These were to be maintained by the Soroptomists. He

[78] Evans, W. 'Check-up Controversy' BMA Swansea 1965, *Daily Telegraph*, 16.7.1965.
[79] Evans, T. 'A Countryman at Heart'. Interview, *Cambrian News*. Dec. 24, 1982.

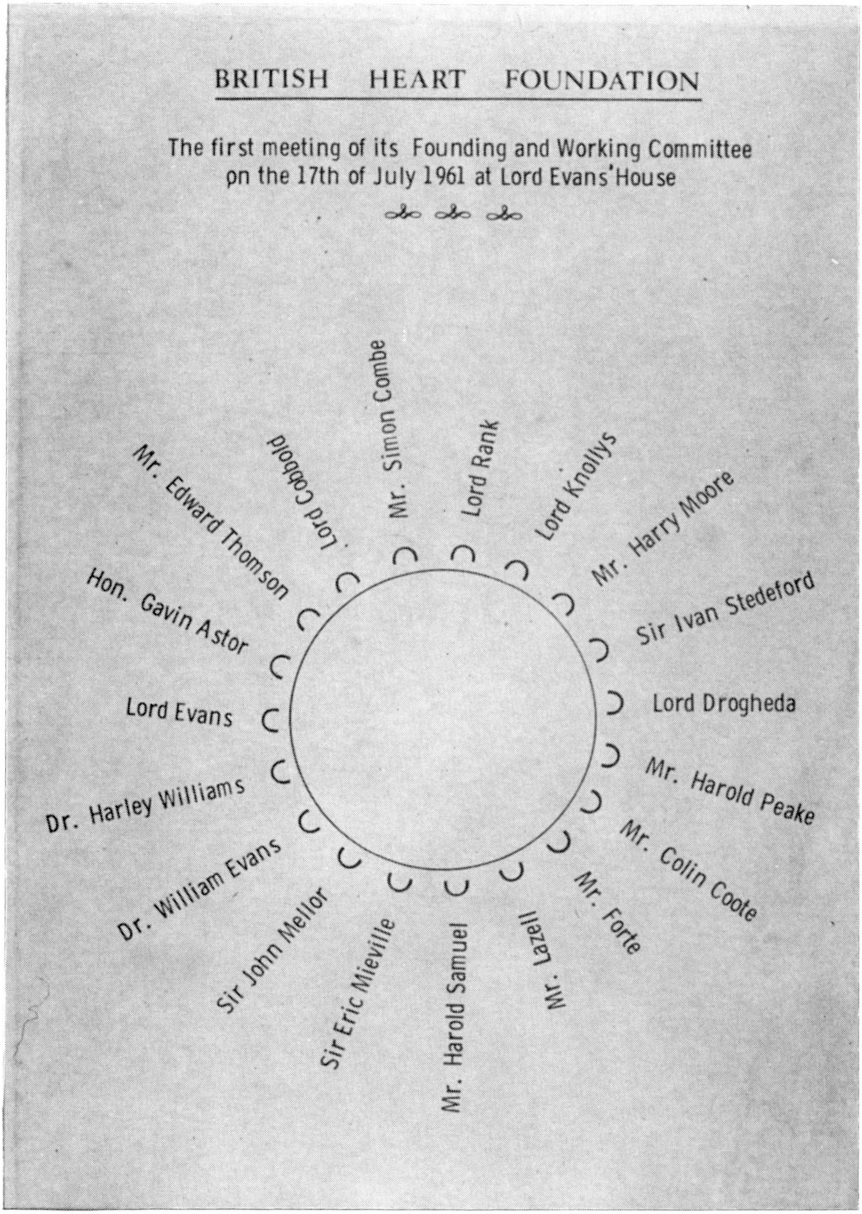

# BRITISH HEART FOUNDATION

The first meeting of its Founding and Working Committee
on the 17th of July 1961 at Lord Evans' House

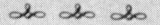

Mr. Simon Combe
Lord Rank
Lord Cobbold
Lord Knollys
Mr. Edward Thomson
Mr. Harry Moore
Hon. Gavin Astor
Sir Ivan Stedeford
Lord Evans
Lord Drogheda
Dr. Harley Williams
Mr. Harold Peake
Dr. William Evans
Mr. Colin Coote
Sir John Mellor
Mr. Forte
Sir Eric Mieville
Mr. Lazell
Mr. Harold Samuel

British Heart Foundation Dinner at Lord Evans' home.
*(Photograph by permission of Miss Frances Evans.)*

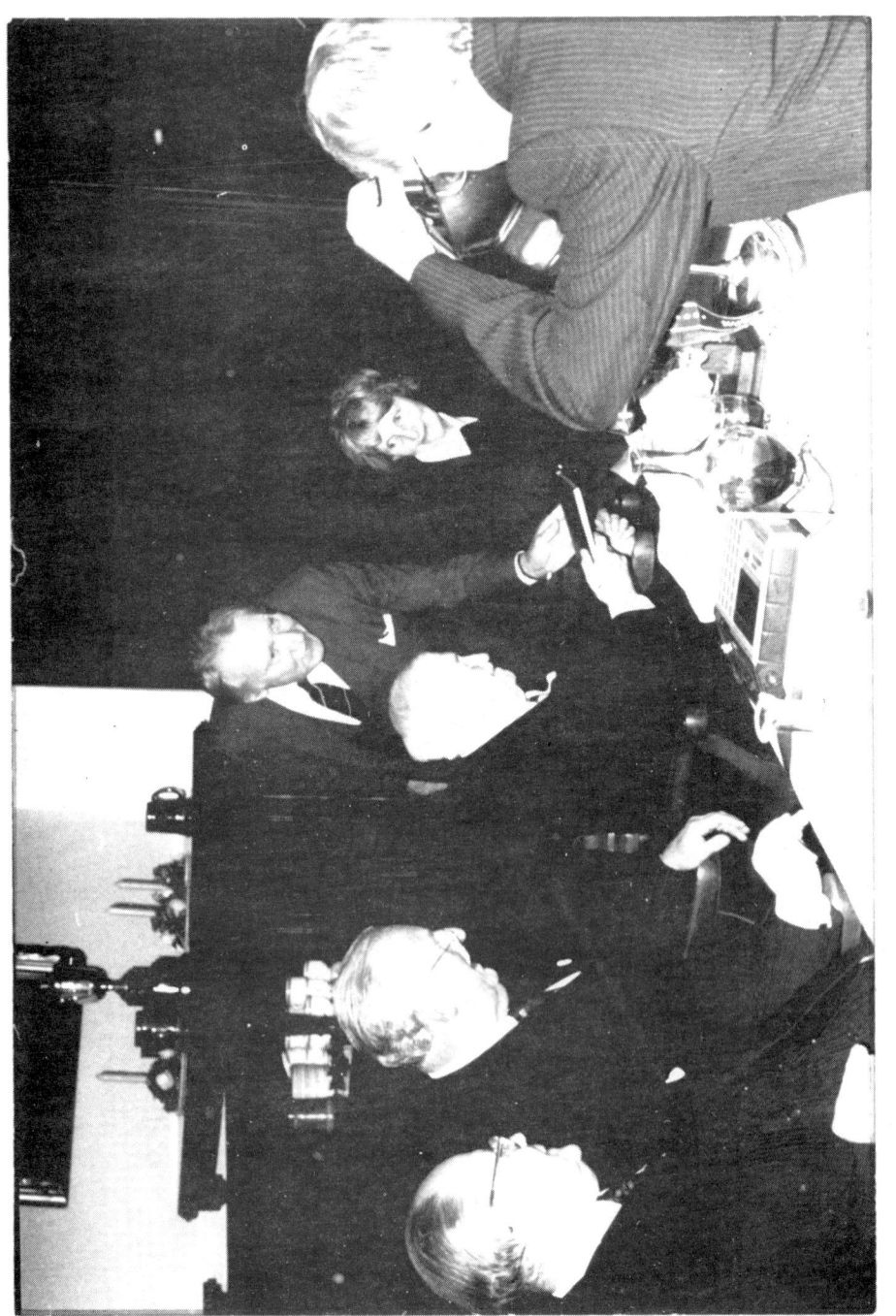

Birthday Party at 90.

*Left to Right:* Roderic Bowen, Byron Evans, William Evans, Frances Evans, Wallace Brigden (standing).

*(Photograph by permission of Miss Frances Evans.)*

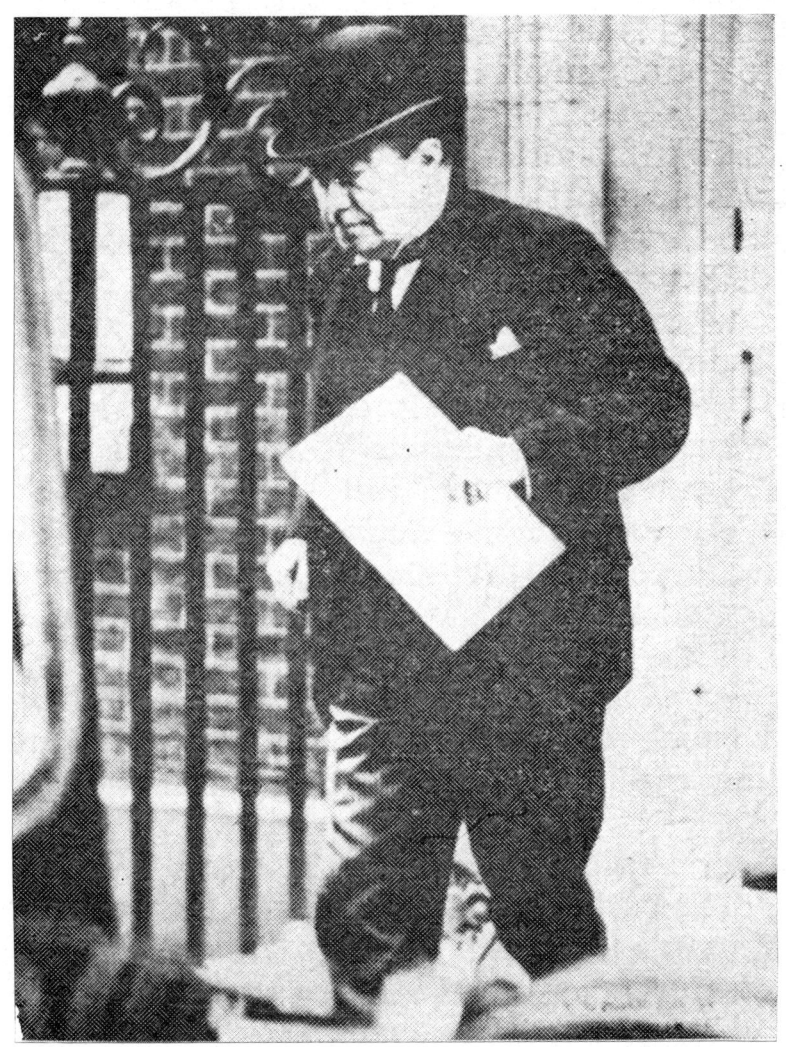

Baldwin.
*(Photograph by permission of Miss Frances Evans.)*

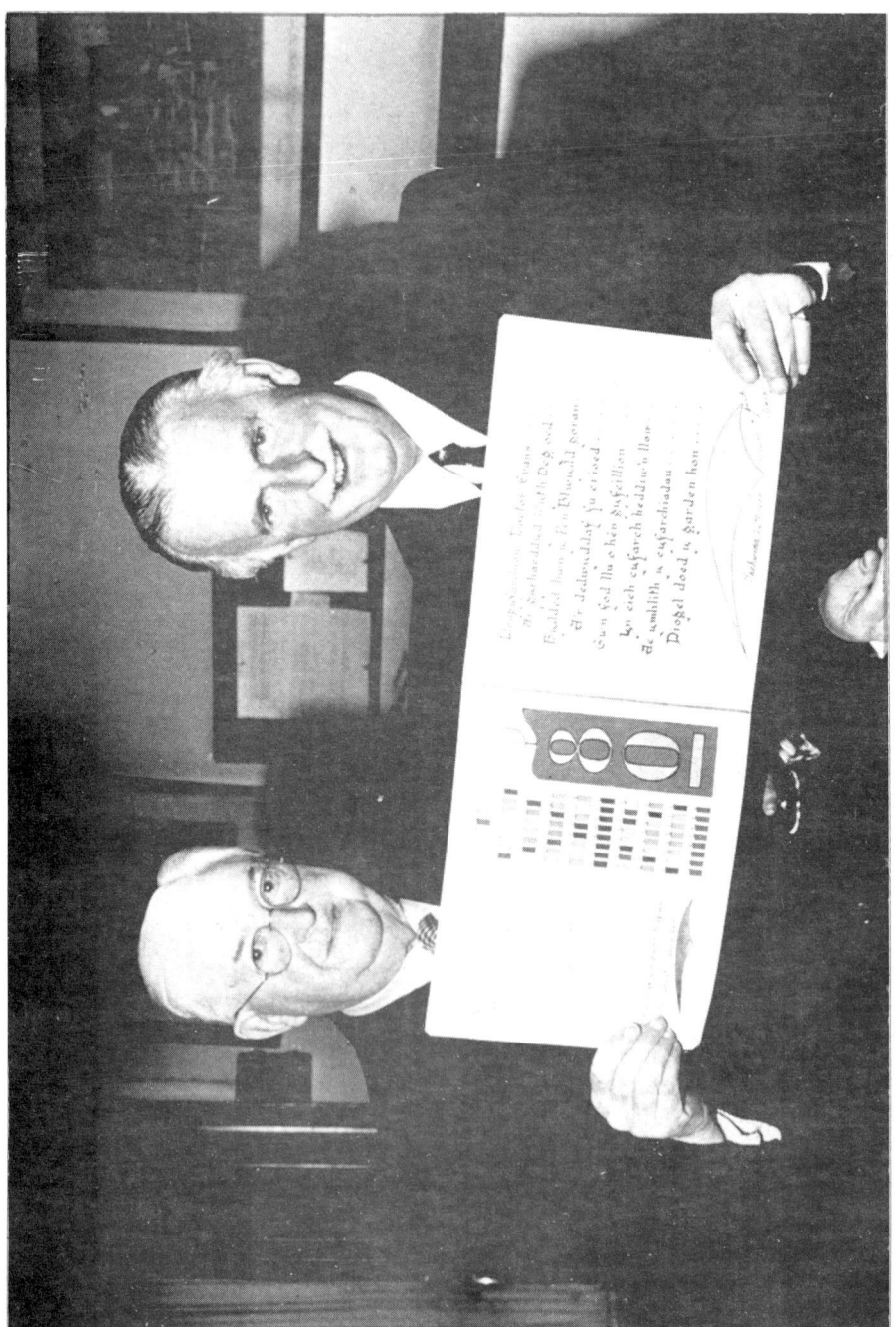

With Byron Evans at 80th Birthday Party.
*(Photograph by permission of Miss Frances Evans.)*

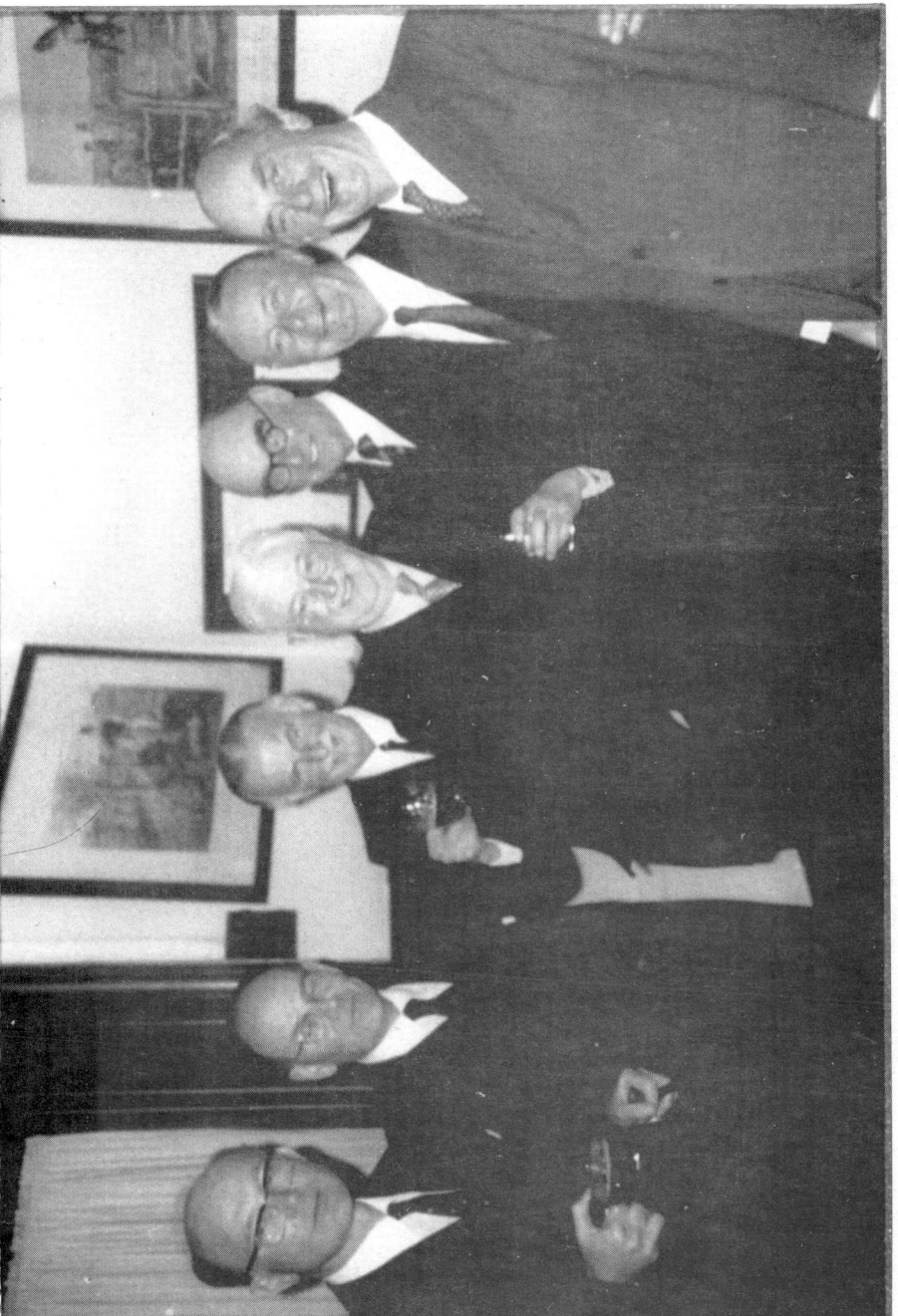

Birthday Party at 80.

*(Photograph by permission of Miss Frances Evans.)*

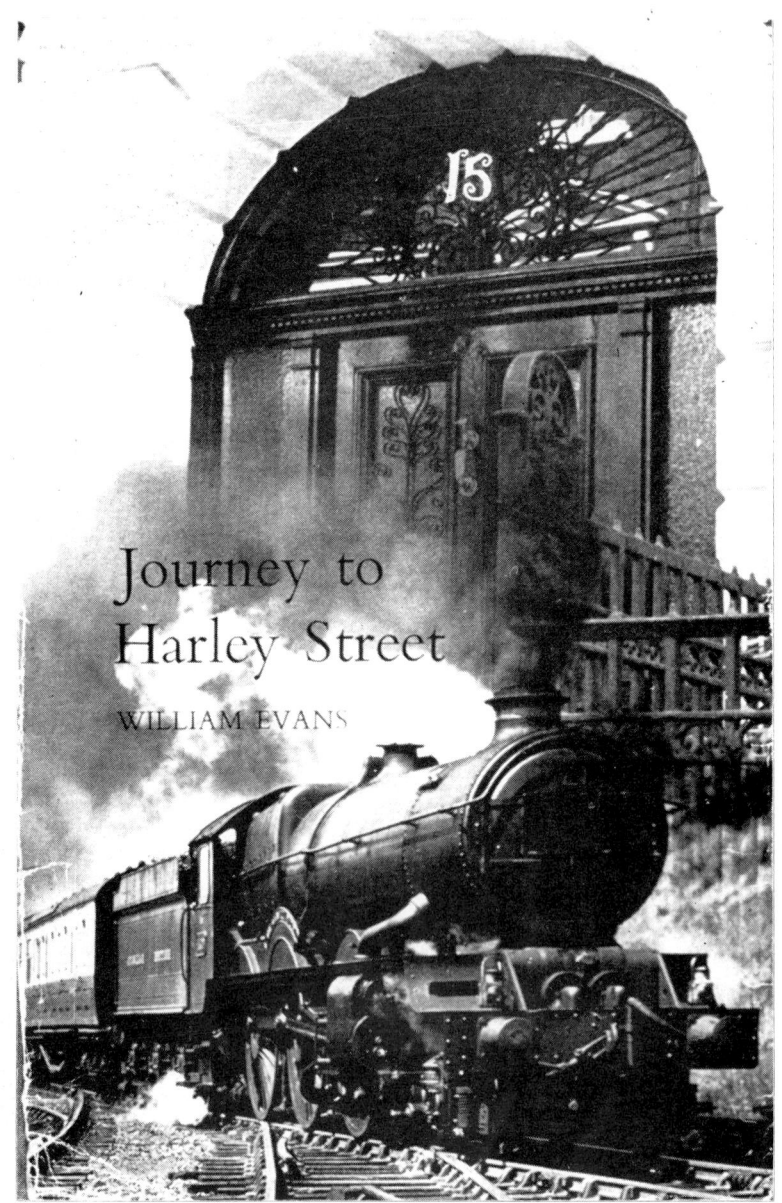

Journey to
Harley Street

WILLIAM EVANS

Cover illustration of Autobiography.
*(Photograph by permission of Miss Frances Evans.)*

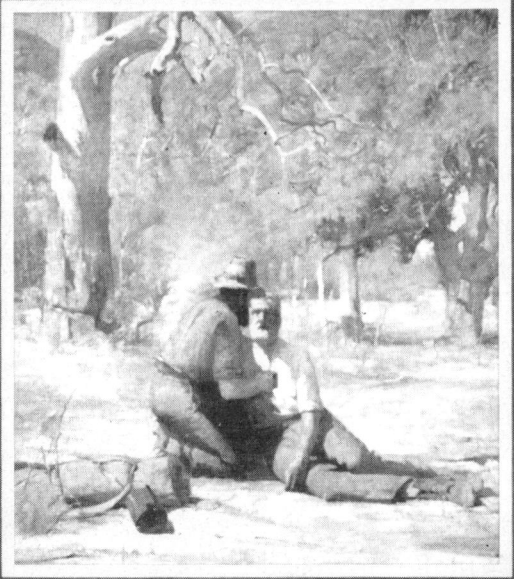

Diary of a Welsh Swagman.
*(Photograph by permission of Miss Frances Evans.)*

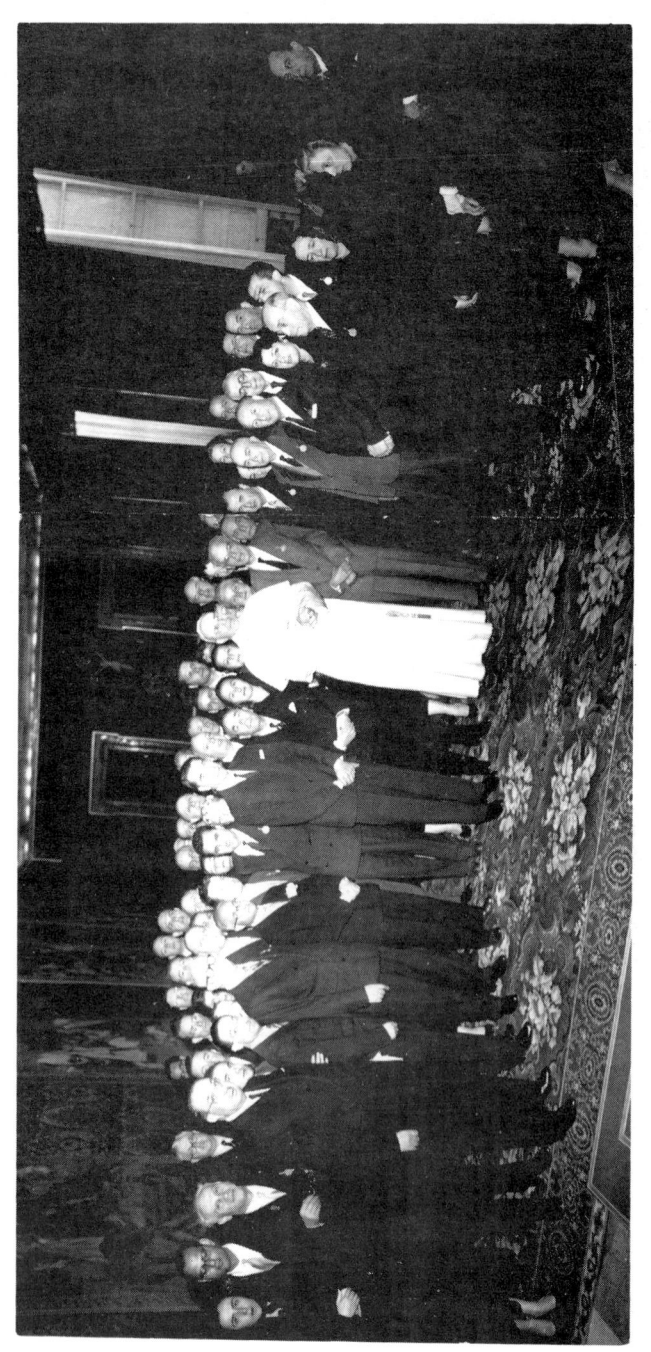

An Audience with His Holiness Pope Pius XII, 1956.
(WE fourth from left).

*(Photograph by permission of Miss Frances Evans.)*

responded generously to the many voluntary organisations who asked him for assistance.

On his 90th birthday he was given another party by his old assistants with an Album with the inscription

> William Evans on your 90th Birthday 24 November 1985 a few of your Friends, Colleagues and Students were privileged to be present at the Cardiff and County Club in your Honour.
> We are grateful to you for your help, guidance, wise counsel, and teaching over many years. rest assured that you will always be remembered with deep affection and respect by us all'.

He wore the tie of the Lancashire Fusiliers at the Party and although he was very frail he spoke to his many friends and associates and made a speech to thank them for coming. The list of old Londoners present was published in the *London Hospital Gazette*.

One of his maxims was 'to pave the last mile one needs spiritual resiliency'.

Then on a long life he quoted:– 'It has been said that :– "a long life is like a long dinner except the sweets come first. Yet after the sweets come the savoury and it is the long-lived that can savour best through memory, the refineries of life".

He also quotes William Hunter on his death bed: 'If I had strength to hold a pen, I would write how easy and pleasant a thing it is to do'.

He was not afraid of death, 'The fear of death is greater torment than dying and death is like sleeping only longer'.

In an Epilogue to a review of Hospices – 'O Lord support us all the day long' (Prayer Book 1662) WE said, 'Surely that is the quintessence of hospice care'.

In the *Times* of 1967 he is quoted as suggesting that there should be wardens to look after the old and disabled. When Dr Eluned Woodford Williams had arrived at Tregaron Hospital to make an inspection of the hospital, WE had been summoned to lunch with her and they got the Health Authority to change their plans to close the Hospital but instead to build another wing to care for short-stay and convalescing patients. This faces Tyndomen and was officially opened by Professor John Petty in June 1982.

In 1965 he had written a booklet for the Chest and Heart Association, called 'Need I ever retire?' giving his philosophy and advocating work. He described the idle as a peculiar kind of dead who can not be buried. 'Plan for Retirement and fill your day. Share the chores, read, write and take outdoor activity'. This was a modern approach.

Minerva in the BMJ remembered him with affection and almost with awe on behalf of generations of students to whom he taught cardiology. She also remembered his compassion and his emphasis on the importance of a good education for socially deprived children with rheumatic heart disease who would be ill-suited to manual work.

In the 90th birthday Album his friends and associates had written their tributes:–

Michael Floyer, London:

> You are 90 and the College 200 at the same time. Many thanks for all the help, advice and teaching which you have given me during the last 44 years.

Arthur Hollman, London:

> Your devotion to teaching will never be forgotten and neither will your devotion to Digitalis.

Frederick Jackson, West Chinock:

> Have you got your books?
> Have you got it down?
> You, have you? – well cross it out.

He loved living in Bryndomen and had a lot of visitors, medical friends from far and wide as well as locals. Frances would act as hostess but he loved entertaining, bread and butter pudding being a favourite. He had a time table which he wrote out beforehand and was very methodical.

He died on 20 September 1988, was cremated, and his ashes placed with Christina's in Marylebone Crematorium.

A service of thanksgiving for his life was held in St. Caron's Church on 22 October 1988. A simple moving service taken by the young vicar Rev. Edward J. Lewis and an address given by Professor Michael Floyer formerly Dean of the London Hospital Medical College. The first lesson Sirach 38, v. 1-10 & 12-15, 'Honour the Physician with Honour due to him; according to your need of him' was read by Dr Hugh Herbert and the 2nd lesson from St. Luke's Gospel 8, v. 41 to the end by his nephew Dr Ebben Roderic-Evans.

Chapter 10

# Vignettes & De Senectute

After retirement and his return to Tregaron he gave talks and wrote papers on Vignettes of the past and De Senectute (Old Age)[80] which were published in *The British Medical Journal*. Cicero was only 64 when he wrote De Senectute (About Old Age). This had been a Latin set-book when WE was in school but he considered that Cicero had not enough experience of life at that age to do the subject justice. He felt one needed to be older and have close associates who are older. He asks 'is it a granary of accumulated wisdom or a depleted grist of lost opportunities'? He considered life to have three phases – child, adult and 'you look wonderful'. The hair can be tinted and cosmetics can work wonders for the face so the hands are the best clue to age. He advocated a weekly hair-do for women to keep up appearances and thought it better than tablets to boost morale. A quiet place to meditate and work to occupy oneself was essential and he quotes Alexander Pope:–

Want of occupation is not rest, a mind quite vacant is a mind distressed'.

The infirmities of old age have to be dealt with as does loneliness following bereavement. For insomnia he advocated a tot of whisky and as for diet 'a little of what you fancy does you good'. At the end, death is a journey into the unknown and an insoluble puzzle which we need not fear for death is like sleep only longer. He believed, as was St. David's prayer, that God would not cast him out when he was old and he believed in the immortality of the soul. After the article appeared in the BMJ he received thanks for his words of wisdom, joy and courage.

Serendip[81] was the former name of Ceylon now Sri Lanka and Horace Walpole narrated a fairy tale of 'The Three Princes of

[80] Evans, W. 'De Senectute' BMJ, 1981, Vol.283, p. 1642-1650.
[81] Evans, W. 'Chance, Coincidence, Serendipity' *BMJ*, 1979. Vol. 2 p. 847.

Serendip' whereby three heroes discovered by accident or their own sagacity repeated discoveries. In the history of medicine chance often played a part in diagnosis, aetiology or treatment of disease. In Serendipity there are two factors; that of chance observation and the vision of the observer.

His chief Dr Lewis Smith[82] compared the murmur of aortic regurgitation as 'ruff-duff' to the noise produced by a steam engine in Cambridge Heath Station. During the war he was in a train going from Essex to Liverpool Street Station which was diverted and at one station when it stopped he became aware of 'ruff-duff' from the engine and enquiry revealed the station was Cambridge Heath – a coincidence of verifying the station with the sound.

In another when he was demonstrating a rare Dovecote murmur from a rupture of an Aortic cusp as 'woo-woo' a pigeon seated on a railing outside the open window replied 'woo-woo'.

A sister discovered a very loud noise coming from her brother's chest which was 'woo' – a ruptured mitral valve.

He recounted the tale of a chance teaparty[83] when a woman with anaemia met a Nursing Sister from the London Hospital who advised her to eat lightly cooked liver each day. This was a long time before Drs Minot & Murphy had discovered this but he was unable to find out the identity of the Sister who had made the comment.

In April 1964 he was invited to talk to business executives in London and told them that exercise was good for the heart. The following day his wife was lunching in Harrods and was joined by a lady who told her she had read this advice in the *Daily Telegraph*[84] and had decided to walk to Harrods feeling immediate benefit. A coincidence to be telling his wife the story.

He remembered a local fisherman[85] in his youth who had an emergency amputation of a leg following a compound fracture of the femur which resulted in the end of the femur projecting 3/4″ through the flesh. What fascinated him as a child was to see maggots falling from the end of the femur when he discarded his peg leg. Years later in pre-penicillin days Professor Trueta of Spain and later of Oxford used a poultice of maggots to deal with inflammation of bone.

[82] Evans, W. 'Heart murmurs mimicked' *BMJ*, 1980. No. 6219. Vol. 280, p. 1006.
[83] Evans, 'A tea-party in Derbyshire' BMJ, 1979. No. 6198. Vol. 2, p. 1123.
[84] Evans, W. 'A ready believer gets it partly right', BMJ, 1980. Vol. 281, p. 1131.
[85] Evans, W. 'Maggots galore', BMJ, 1979. No. 6194. Vol. 2, p. 847.

On one occasion a clairvoyant[86] willed that he should have a pain in his neck for what she considered a broken promise during her treatment and at the precise time he had a severe attack of torticollis which lasted several hours. Was this a coincidence or proof of the existence of telepathic transmission? For some time afterwards he had a lurking respect for the cult of clairvoyancy.

An amazing tale was of a visit by Sir Robert Hutchinson[87] to a patient in the East End who was baffled for a diagnosis in a lady with fever and delirium, when a tug on his coat by a child of eight told him 'I know what is wrong with Auntie, she's got what the parrot died of'. The patient was admitted to hospital and examined by the Pathologist, Dr Samuel Bedson who indeed discovered and described the virus of Psittocosis. For this work Bedson was awarded a knighthood – following the chance remark by a child.

The presence of accessory nipples[88] increases the risk of genetic or congenital connotation. He discovered accessory nipples (polythelia) in a patient with pulmonary hypertension and a week later found a second patient with both so decided to seek polythelia in each patient who came to see him for any reason. When he had 2000 cases he analysed his findings and found the incidence of polythelia in the healthy group to be 5%. In the diseased group with congenital heart disease he found an accessory nipple in 14%. In two conditions cardiomyopathy and pulmonary hypertension the figure was near 44%. In a group of hypertensive patients 35% had polythelia who also had left ventricular hypertrophy (LVH).

In another hypertensive group without LVH only 5% had polythelia. This study supports the classification of hypertension into true hypertension where the ECG shows LVH and another of hypertonia where the ECG is normal. He makes the case that it is important to differentiate between them as the first group needs treatment and the second should not be subjected to invalidism and unnecessary prescribing of symptom producing drugs.

The finding of two young brothers[89] both of whom were supposedly healthy who were found to have enlarged hearts and died suddenly made him examine other members of the family. Their mother, two

[86] Evans, W. 'A clairvoyant practises her cult', BMJ, 1980. No. 6213. Vol. 280, p. 551.
[87] Evans, W. 'Wisdom from the infant's mouth'. BMJ, 1979 . No. 6198. Vol. 2. p. 1123.
[88] Evans, W. 'A surface sign with deep meaning.' BMJ, 1979, No. 6197. Vol. 2. p. 1058.
[89] Evans, W. 'Like breeds like' BMJ, 1979, Vol. 6196. Vol. 2. p. 986.

aunts and uncle had died suddenly and their maternal grandparents had died aged 30. He named the condition Familial Cardiomegaly in a communication in 1949.

It was the chance persistence of a student[90] who found an abnormal ECG in a patient with Friedereich's Ataxia whose brother had the same combination of findings which sparked his interest in collecting cases of Friedereich's Ataxia from other hospitals and 38 patients found. He wrote a joint paper with George Wright the student on Friederich's Ataxia in 1942 showing the heart was affected as well as the central nervous system in this disease.

Only rarely had heart failure been recorded in Friedreich's Ataxia since Newton Pitts case in 1987. He recounts the tale of Oliver[91] who had this syndrome and was in a home for incurables but who spent time as an inpatient either at Guy's or the London Hospital and both Physicians were anxious to examine his Spinal Cord when he died. He died in Guy's but when the London physicians asked to see the notes they were told that they had been destroyed. Later WE was given a copy of the autobiography of Sir Arthur Hurst, a physician of Guy's, who had been house physician to Newton Pitt and in it discovered that when the post-mortem on Oliver had been carried out, the Spinal Cord was removed but a gush of water took it into the drain from where it was not retrieved so the examination of a Spinal Cord with this disease had to wait for another patient.

Eirian Williams[92] one of WE's old students recounts the afternoon in 1945 when two young students were being questioned by WE in the outpatient clinic. WE questioned one on the polygraph and its inventor Sir James Mackenzie. To each question the student knew the answer of what Sir James had done before going to the London; where he had lived and what the plaque above the door said. At the end WE asked the student how he knew so much about Mackenzie to be told that the student's father had taken over his practice when Sir James moved to London and he was born in Sir James' old consulting room. Serendipitous?

Another problem recounted was the chance finding of a parathyroid tumour in a policeman[93] who died from pneumonia following

[90] Evans, W. 'The persistent student' *BMJ*, 1979, No. 6195. Vol. 2, p. 930.
[91] Evans, W. 'The lost cord' *BMJ*, 1980, Vol. 281. p. 786.
[92] Williams, E., 'Chance, coincidence, serendipity' – 'The biter bit' *BMJ*, 1980. Vol. 281. p. 1190.
[93] Evans, W. 'P. C. Mulvaney' *BMJ*, 1979 No. 6195. Vol. 2. p. 930.

spontaneous fracture of the femur in decalcified bone. Twenty one years later when WE was Registrar to Dr Donald Hunter he was researching Calcium metabolism and looking up old records of patients who had similar fractures. At this time a man was admitted with a history of multiple fractures whom Dr Hunter suspected of having a parathyroid tumour and persuaded a surgeon to operate when indeed a tumour was found. It was luck that the policeman had fallen outside the London Hospital and that his post-mortem should have been carried out by Dr H. M. Turnbull, later Professor of the Faculty and a Fellow of the Royal Society.

Another interesting item appeared in Materia Non Medica in the BMJ which he recalled as Bibliomedical similitude.[94] This was a quotation he heard on a radio programme Quote – Unquote and that night read by chance in his Bible, Deuteronomy 10th Chapter 16v. – 'Circumcise therefore the foreskin of your heart and be no more stiff-necked' spoken by Moses to the Israelites before entering the promised land. This verse alludes to treatment – the surgical treatment of constrictive pericarditis. He had often discussed this treatment with his surgical colleagues Tudor Edwards, Donald Barlow, and Vernon Thompson when they had emphasised the importance of removing all the adhesive material to the atrioventricular groove which would be a circumcision. The term 'stiff-necked' was related to dyspnoea associated with the feeling of tightness of the neck not heart failure. These facts reveal that the surgical treatment was outlined in Mosaic Law and had remained hidden for 2000 years until revealed on a Radio Parlour game. An example of the long arm of coincidence.

In 1983 he reviewed a book on life in a Welsh Valley by Francis Maylett Smith called *The Surgery at Aberffrwd: some encounters of a Colliery Doctor*.[95] It highlights the mediocrity and dormancy of medicine during the first part of this century, progress in diagnosis and treatment in the middle and as we enter the New Century, we should stand studiously still as we contemplate further progress , avoiding unwarranted and invasive investigations of the patients, refraining from adopting adventurous therapeutic procedures, medical or surgical, born of curiosity or lust and as yet not adjudged to produce consistent hazard-free benefit. He advocates avoiding unnecessary investigations and adventurous therapeutic procedures.

[94] Evans, W. Bibliomedical similitude *BMJ*, 1979 Vol. 1. p. 1617.
[95] Evans, W. 'Life in a Welsh Valley'. Review of 'The Surgery at Aberffrwd'. *BMJ*, 1983. Vol. 286. p.1035-1036.

Chapter 11

# Diary of a Welsh Swagman 1869-1894

WE's grandfather, Joseph Jenkins lived and worked as a Swagman in Australia for 25 years;[96] a swagman being a vagrant worker who carried his personal possessions in a pack or swag while travelling about in search of work.

During his life he wrote fifty-eight diaries; thirty-three about his life in Wales and twenty-five whilst in Australia. Joseph had seen that the diaries which were bulky were returned to Wales and given to his daughter Nel, where they remained in the attic of her home in Tyndomen until WE was encouraged to publish them by Dr Thomas Paxton of Adelaide. They have become an Australian classic; the first edition published in 1975 and since reprinted six times. Nel had bequeathed them to her grand-daughter Frances and the Welsh diaries are now in the National Library of Wales Aberystwyth and the Australian diaries in the State Library of Victoria in Melbourne.

He had started writing a diary in order to improve his command and usage of English and to be able to correspond in the language, using a quill pen with ink, never a pencil. Even during long tiring days in Australia when he would have to get up at 3.30 to 4 a.m. in order to go ploughing he would only go to bed after writing his diary; often as late as 10 p.m. The first diaries were in books and later note paper 8″ by 5″ which he bound with thick brown twine and covered with thick brown paper or linen.

In 1857 his home farm Trecefel was the best in the county of Cardiganshire where he practised a rotational system for growing crops, grew lucerne and clover for animal feed, and fed the soil with farmyard manure. He advised landowners on the drainage and reclamation of land and animal husbandry and those who sought his advice included Powell of Nanteos, Davies of Llandinam and Lord Lisburne so he held a position of authority in the community. He

[96] Evans, W. Diary of a Welsh Swagman.

72

excelled in hedging, ploughing, scything, ditching and thatching. He advised on construction of dykes for irrigation and transport and on the siting of bridges when the railway was constructed.

Why did he decide to emigrate when he was 51 years old? The probable reason was the deteriorating relationship with his wife. In his diary for December 1892 there is a press cutting 'A man asks a magistrate what to do with a disagreeable wife – leave her'!

In 1876 he had written in his diary 'It was my fault I absented myself from my home'. Bethan Phillips in her book about him *Rhwng Dau Fyd* blames alcohol and consorting with the wealthy for his deterioration and lack of control of his farm and finances. He had probably chosen Australia as he had heard of the Goldrush and thought he would have no difficulty getting work with his skills.

He left Trecefel without telling anyone, at night, taking the train from Aberystwyth to Liverpool on 8 December 1868. He arrived at Port Melbourne on 22 March 1869. His diaries give an unique account of Colonial Australia where he worked on farms in the Ballarat and Castlemain area and later as a street worker involved with drains for Maldon Council.

He was an unusual Swagman to say the least and became concerned with land degradation, cruelty to animals, the treatment of Aboriginals and the increasing unemployment spreading amongst farm workers with resulting high suicide rate.

He needed fortitude to withstand his isolated hard lonely deprived life and courage to endure the illness and hardship he encountered. He had Welsh friends who befriended him and he enjoyed local Eisteddfodau where he won prizes for his poems. He wrote these in English and Welsh and 80 were published in *Cerddi Cerngoch*. He read the Bible every day and enjoyed the Classics. In 1884 he read Pope's translation of Homer's Iliad and commented in the diary 'the composition was so good'.

WE's purpose in sharing the diaries with the public was twofold. He felt it was clearly his grandfather's wish that his thoughts be shared with others and it stands as a testament to the early days of the Colony. It is a classic story in Joseph's own words which has been sensitively abridged by WE and is now one of the subjects used in the school curriculum in Australia.

To get the full flavour one needs to read the book but I shall draw out some of the medical aspects for the reader.

Joseph took a medical chest with him from Liverpool and two years after his arrival in Australia wrote that it now contained only Cayenne Pepper and Eye-water. His Laudanum bottle had broken. This he had used on four occasions and had found it useful. He had also run out of Quinine. He mentions Laudanum medication 20-50 drops for Dysentery several times in the Diary. The Cayenne Pepper had been used to disperse colic and he noted that it also warmed his feet. He had used it externally as a cure and treatment for snake bite. He treated a second attack of Quinsy with it and in 1880 bad colds with a mixture of Cayenne Pepper, Salt, Senna, Ginger and Sugar dissolved in a pint of warm beer. As he was no better the following day he repeated the mixture in a quart of beer and immersed his feet in mustard and water though again to no avail.

For rheumatism which started in 1871 he took more mustard with his meat.

There is an account of his weekly shopping list for 1873 which came to 12s-4d and included two loaves, 12lbs meat, 2lbs sugar, potatoes 14lbs, Medicine: though he does not say what this was as salt, pepper, tobacco and mustard are mentioned separately. Newspapers cost 6d. and wear and tear of tools and clothes 2s.

By the end of 1886 and a long period of Dysentery which left him weak, anorexic and depressed he writes that he is tired of meat and potatoes and his favourite meal is oatmeal in milk or bread in boiled milk. He drinks beef tea and eats eggs. By January 1887 he is eating 3lbs. sugar a week and later in the diary he takes sugar in water for energy when unwell.

He had several illnesses necessitating hospital admission.

In July 1874 he was taken desperately ill with Quinsy and Diphtheria and was admitted to Maryborough Hospital at Majorca for forty days. His diary continues with complaints of the rigidity of hospital discipline, his bed was too far from the fireplace, and the open windows resulted in draughts, the beds were too close together and the nights were disturbed by the coughs and groans of others. He felt better sitting in a chair but the rules prevented this.

By September he was staying with a friend and though he visited the doctor several times he had no treatment of benefit and was told by him that he was a chronic and hopeless case.

Obviously the doctor did not know of WE's maxim that no patient should be worse from seeing the doctor! At this time he was complaining of such weakness of his hands and feet that he could not button or unbutton his coat and a month later he was admitted to Inglewood Hospital for a month presumably to convalesce.

In October 1878 he entered Ballarat Hospital to a ward of thirty patients and underwent a most painful operation when an injection was made into the base of his bladder which left him in agony, unable to walk and hardly able to stand. He makes a pertinent statement, 'It appears to me that for the sake of comfort and improved health the patients are confined to bed for too long a time. To keep men in bed day and night when they are able and anxious to get up and walk through the garden is indefensible'. This was a century before this became common practice.

He had a second operation which was not so painful and was in hospital for 18 days in all. However, he continued to remain unwell and in pain with blood in his urine and wrote 'I am in a most inconvenient place to die – 15 miles from the cemetery'.

He was admitted to Castlemaine Hospital in November and wrote 'My body begins to swell. I would like to see my children once more'. He was discharged in December and walked eight miles to a friend's house in this weakened state. He must have continued to feel ill for he made a Will. In May 1890 he is admitted to hospital with Dysentery but by October is better than he has been for years.

Toothache is a recurring theme in the Diary and by December 1883 he had a new set of dentures. However in 1892 toothache in a remaining stump had to be endured as he comments that 'Doctors in Australia are deadly reckless'. One cure for toothache is to soak cotton wool in best brandy and put in the ear of the affected side!

He had several accidents through his work. In April 1875 a chip of wood flew into his left eye while he was chopping it and gave him a sore eye and loss of half his vision in that eye. In 1879 he mentions his sore eye and in 1881 he got a 'Sandy Blight' in one of his eyes. This is a very small poisonous fly and his eye was closed by swelling in two hours.

In May 1876 he was kicked in the thigh by a colt which became very painful. In 1880 'whilst drawing water from a well the handle of the winch slipped as it spun at high speed and hit me on the forehead. I was stunned and fell across the platform and narrowly missed falling into the well which is 70´ deep'.

In 1882 he writes that he is harassed by worms, ants and flies. In 1887 he fell and was thought to have fractured two ribs as he had difficulty in breathing. The doctor put a plaster on his side and told him not to work for a long time – he went to work the next day!

In 1888 he injured his right fore-finger which became stiff and in order to be able to write he had to tie his middle finger to it. Writing remained difficult as noted in 1890. In that year he scalded his feet which became swollen, oozed from broken blisters and he was not able to bear weight.

He wrote that he had several escapes from death during his life, his 7th narrow escape in 1881 occurred when a stack of hay weighing four tons fell over and he only just managed to get out of its way.

A letter from his daughter Nel which he received in November 1890 told him his grandson Ieuan had died and that his brother Benjamin had been in bed with consumption for two months. He later reads in a paper cutting of Benjamin's death. He was a Solicitor aged 51, the youngest of his parents twelve children. Joseph was very fond of him and cried at the news.

In 1891 as a precaution against sunstroke he soaked a piece of calico in water and wrapped it round his head and placed a green cabbage leaf inside his hat. There are several references to family and friends.

In December 1879 he read in the *Aberystwyth Observer* that his daughter Elinor (Nel), WE's mother, had married on the 9th June one of the sons of Crynfrynbychan and that they have gone to farm at Tyndomen. In July 1983 he heard that his eldest daughter Margaret had died on 29.4.1883 aged 32 years.

In September 1887 he read in the *Cambrian News* that his daughter Anne had won a prize at her school in Kensington, London. 'Well done Anne!' – he wrote. Also that his youngest son John David had qualified as a doctor which he read in the *Daily News*. He later had a letter from John letting him know that he was a Doctor of Medicine of the University of London.

In 1889 he reads that his grandson Ieuan Evans, aged 7 (Nel's son and WE's brother) had died.

In 1892 he heard that his daughter Jane had married and later his nephew Jenkin Jenkins (Aeronian) had died aged 46 years. Jenkin had written to him earlier urging him to return home and when he heard of his death and the earlier death of his wife he felt he would like to see their children.

In June 1893 he wrote to Nel and his other married daughter to tell them for the first time since going to Australia that he would like to see his grandchildren.

He writes of undesirable dreams and of his longing to return to Wales.

Even though life was hard he was able to liven it over the years with taking part in literary competitions and reading to enhance his knowledge. In March 1878 he entered a Competition for the best 'Englyn' on Stanley who was at the time exploring the Nile and his was the successful entry in the competition out of six.

His diaries reveal an interest in Phrenology, Voltaire, the philosopher Zorvaster whose advice he followed – 'when a man is in doubt whether to do this or that, the safest plan is to leave it undone!'

In 1881 he wrote that work is life's principal comfort and expressed his gratitude to his parents for compelling him to work when young.

He was interested in Queen Victoria and was three months and three days older than her as she had her birthday on May 24th. In May 1883 he wrote to her to offer his condolences on the death of her faithful servant and intimate friend John Brown.

Towards the end life became increasingly difficult. In January 1892 there was a drought and the temperature was 112°F in the shade. The wind removed part of his roof and he had to have help to mend the damage. He had to walk 400 yards to get water from a water hole and carried it by balancing two kerosene tins containing 11½lbs. on a beam across his shoulders like a chinaman, this when he was 74 years old.

In 1893 when he was complaining of increasing tiredness on walking; his duties as an overseer of water ways covered 40 miles of channels in an area of a square mile. In March he had hiccup which he wrote was a bad sign in an old man and for chronic Dysentery he took 50 drops of Laudanum. In May he was upset that his brother John had died and gave a months notice to the Council as he hoped to sail for Wales in a few months but by June/July he was sorry he had done so as he has a two month wait for a passage. During this year there are several records of his desire to see his grandchildren and that his money was running out. Although he was owed £200 he was unable to collect his debts or sell his property.

On 23 November he went by rail to Melbourne and procured a cabin on the Ophir of Orient Shipping for £26-13-6d and sailed on the 25th. He arrived in Tilbury, London on the 5 January 1895 the journey having taken 41 days in contrast to 193 days it had taken to go out 25 years earlier. He was met by his sons Tom and John, his brother Jenkin and two friends and was asked by Jenkin whether it was indeed he as he had gone from being sturdy and strong to a feeble and tired old man. Days later they returned to Trecefel where he lived until his death on 26 September 1898 aged 80 years.

WE admired 'his abiding philosophy under adverse circumstances, unyielding cheerfulness in the face of disappointments, compassion in lending money from his poor wages to those worse off than himself, his optimism and his faith in the permanence of Nature. The physical work he undertook was hard and towards the end of his time in Australia he was handicapped by declining health and old age'.

His epitaph which he wrote in 1890 reads

> Marw sydd raid, nis gwyddom pryd,
> Pa fodd, pa fan, yn hyn o fyd.
> Ac os iw bywyd i ni'n rhodd,
> Mae marw hefyd yr un modd.
> Can's beth fo'n rhan, mae'n eithaf eglir,
> Cawn chwareu teg gan Awdur Natur.

WE's translation is of a

> A philosophy which accepts our fate
> Die we must, and cast aside this mortal shell,
> How or when and in what place, we cannot tell.
> If we assign to life a gift so rare,
> Then death itself claims equal share,
> Whate'er our fate, it is quite clear,
> We'll get fair-play from earth's Creator.

Willie had inscribed a copy of 'The Swagman' to a friend as follows

William Evans
July 1979                            Gyda chofion gwresog.

within the cover of this book
The reader will find a Treasury of –
> Self-discipline
> Self-reliance, and
> Self-containment.
> W.E.

Chapter 12

# Unanswered Question

A simple countryman with few worldly needs who had found spiritual contentment; he was as happy to mix with his Tregaron friends as he was with his many illustrious friends who called regularly to see him. Professionally he had given generously to his patients, pupils, and medical science.

His first ambition was to be a country doctor in Cefn Gwlad (rural area) but 'I would be no good unless I was surrounded by apparatus – I could only do half a job' he said.

I was told that he was not a physiologist or scientist yet he had gained a D.Sc. in one University and been honoured by a D.Sc. in another! (Appx. II)

In 1931 Dr Thomas Lewis[97] had telephoned WE at the London where he was then a Registrar and invited him to apply for the vacant position of assistant physician at University College Hospital. The local candidate whom Lewis did not regard highly was one of his former assistants. WE remembered the occasion.

'He asked me to meet him to discuss the matter. An appointment was made and I duly attended on a Monday morning at his basement room. When Sir Thomas arrived he took no notice of me, entered his room, sat at his desk and left the door open. Presently I knocked at the door and walked in. I was not invited to take a chair and as I stood before him seated at his desk, he looked up and spoke 'I do not know why you are applying for this post, you have no chance of getting it'. My monkey was up!

I explained that I was doing it at his advice, apologised for interrupting his work and said I was especially sorry to be wasting my own time. I turned to walk away and made for the door. Instantly he was out of his chair and invited me to sit down and we discussed fishing at length'.

[97] Hollman, A. Sir Thomas Lewis. Springer 1997, p. 210-211.

He did not go to UCH!

The British Heart Foundation in their book[97] write that he was always interested in research and helped many young men as assistants in the Department to develop successful careers and some to pursue academic research, Professor Shillingford being one of these. He had received no formal research training himself like most of his contemporaries, and his results were with usage of the results of his clinical experience.

He enthused his juniors who had great affection for him and was a character. Fastidious in dress, professionally meticulous and dedicated to punctuality he was a well-known figure of the national and international scene of the time.

One of his younger colleagues who called to see him in Bryndomen was 10 minutes late and was told so by Willie when he arrived – 'You are 10 minutes late B'![99]

He said of the research worker that he needs patience and perseverance in the face of disappointment. He seeks neither profit, promotion nor self-aggrandisement and earns no reward save satisfaction of having uncovered something to aid ailing fellow-man and what greater reward than this can anyone earn? – None!

For 30 years in clinical consulting practice he gave one day a week to clinical research and had been given good grounding by Professor Turnbull who would go over all research projects with WE when he was writing up his results to make sure that all the sentences were short and crisp.

In a letter[100] to T. G. G. Herbert (Tom) a Vet of Aberaeron on 27 August 76 who had written to congratulate him on becoming a fellow of the Royal Society, he points out the honour is not of course the FRS – 'This was far beyond my reach – but fellow of the Royal Society of Medicine'.

'It came as a surprise to me and I became embarrassed when I found out that among those holding it there is a discoverer of Insulin, discoverer of the principle in the Liver which cures pernicious Anaemia, the joint discoverer of Penicillin, and also the Australian who found the virus of myxomatosis which is introduced to destroy the rabbit.

[98] Mathews, D. N. 'Fighting Heart Disease'. 'The History of the British Heart Foundation' 1961-1988. Blackwell, 1990.
[99] Brigden, W. Personal Information.
[100] Herbert, T. G. G. Papers 22 – National Library, Aberystwyth.

100 are admitted and we are now 91, I am the only Welshman among them and this enhanced my pride on gaining the award'.

During the War the London Hospital Medical School was evacuated to Cambridge and the medical and nursing schools were split. He carried out research in a room next to the kitchens at the London and the evacuation had helped him as it became quiet and easier for recording during Phonocardiography.

Patients under his care were admitted to Orsett Hospital, Essex from the 3rd September 1939 and teaching became disorganised.

Quite early in his career he had seen a man of 64 who had been an invalid all his life because he had been incorrectly diagnosed as a child and he decided to try and prevent this happening in the future by devising what became known as the Essex Scheme. This was early diagnosis of any cardiac condition to prevent invalidism by firstly getting the School Medical Officer to notify the County Medical Officer of Health (MOH) of any cardiac abnormality such as dysrhythmia, murmur or history of rheumatic fever. The MOH would notify the Cardiology Department of the nearest Regional Hospital and the child seen by a Cardiologist. After the diagnosis was made the results would be communicated to the parent, the MOH would notify the Medical Officer, who would tell the teacher; and the General Practitioner. He started this Cardiac Clinic in Oldchurch Hospital in 1941.

He had been appointed Consulting Physician to the Royal Navy and Royal Society of Musicians as well as Messrs. Lloyds Bank and the General Post Office. In 1980 he was elected a 'Knight of Mark Twain' in recognition of his outstanding contribution to modern medical science.

Eirian Williams[101] described his seemingly uncontrived method of teaching as a mixture of dogmatism, challenge and unashamed public oratory. Vows were taken, never to be broken; commandments written down, some to be crossed out. He was an unconventional teacher, effective and entertaining, requiring audience participation and was Free. His most enduring legacy is the gospel of champion of compassion and commonsense in the treatment of disease.

His ever friendly outgoing personality shone as an example to everyone as to how the ideal physician should relate to his patients and students.[102] Senator Hubert Humphrey, Vice President USA quoted

[101] Williams, E. Obituary William Evans. Brit.Med.Jr. 1988. 297, 913-914.
[102] Cooke, B. Personal Information.

WE's paper 'Addiction to Medicines'[103] when he addressed the Senate on Corruption in the Drug Trade, showing his influence infiltrated far and wide. He was not always right but he was a man of great courage who was not afraid to speak as he found things.

He had made an intelligent guess that Dr Martyn Lloyd-Jones' nervousness at a Medical Breakfast was due to the fact that he missed speaking from the pulpit. The subject was 'The Doctor Himself' for which he had prepared his address but at the last moment decided to speak simply on the gospel of the parable of the rich farmer Luke 12 : 13-21.[104] He believed the medical profession had particular temptations, one of the chief being the peril of objectivity. 'I beseech you, do not forget yourself, that you are a man and not merely a doctor'. His message was well received and one which WE stressed to his students.

After he retired in 1960 he remained in Harley Street carrying out his private practice and taking part in Medical Tribunals until he moved to Wales.

In 1967 he spoke in the Royal Naval Hospital, Haslar, in a Symposium on Chest Disease and Allied Disorders on 'Pulmonary Hypertension' a new term for heart failure.[105]

I was told that he did not like women by two separate sources and this surprised me as I had found him charming and he had a happy marriage. He married at 41 years old after gaining professional and financial security and although Christina was 11 years older, theirs was a companionable marriage with mutual interests. I think he was very independent and a private man who could manage Bryndomen by himself when he first retired to Wales, decorating the house, making curtains and hanging them, cooking and painting the fridge instead of buying a new one, showing his true 'Cardi' streak. Frances cared for him during his last feeble years and she told me that he had been very good to her.

He preferred speaking English rather than Welsh but wrote cynghanedd (a form of strict Welsh poetry). He was fond of poetry and literature and quoted from both extensively in his speeches. As a student he had been friendly with T. H. Parry-Williams.[106] His motto

---

[103] Evans, W. 'Addiction to Medicines'. Winchester Division. BMA. Brit.Med.Jr. 1962 ii. p. 722-725.
[104] Murray, I. H. – 'Dr Martyn Lloyd-Jones'. The Banner of Truth Trust. 1990. p. 334-335.
[105] Evans, W. Pulmonary Hypertension – Symposium on Chest Disease, Royal Naval Hospital, Haslar. 25-26 Oct. 1967.
[106] Phillips, B. Personal Information.

for life was Scott's 'Be a Good Man'. Learn and profit from history. Made in Wales should be a sign of star workmanship. Marriage was sacred with duties and responsibilities. Work was valuable and health giving.

At the request of St. Caron's Church Council[107] Tregaron he compiled a booklet on the Church of 15 pages. This was printed by the *Cambrian News* but has no date.

He gives the history of the church which started in the 6th Century with two of its monumental stones now in the National Museum in Cardiff.

The South Chancel window depicts St. Ursula which is of interest to me as Llangwyryfon Church is dedicated to St. Ursula. The wrought iron screen is a gift of the Trecefel family in memory of their nephew John Samuel Jenkins who died aged 20 in 1924.

In Tyndomen, framed, is a quote penned in Calligraphy by Sir William Temple. (See p. 84)

> The greatest pleasure of life is Love
> The greatest treasure contentment
> The greatest possession health
> The greatest ease is Sleep
> The greatest need is a friend.

He was a fortunate man who had many true friends who kept visiting him to the end although he had not socialised much in London.

Amongst his papers was a letter from Sir Henry Cohen[108] in 1955. Sir Henry had invited him to preside over the Section of Medicine of the Joint Meeting of the British and Canadian Associations in Toronto in 1955. Also to give a paper and serve on a panel. The hand written reply from Sir Henry on receiving his acceptance indicated that it was important that Britain be represented by its most distinguished doctors and 'none fills that role better than you'!

A newspaper heading of the event 'Claims Angina Patient should not change jobs but chew glyceryl trinitrate for pain'. About a quarter of the patients diagnosed as Angina turn out to be other ailments such as dyspepsia.

An Editorial[109] in the *British Medical Journal* in 1983 on Chest Pain; heart or gullet? points out that a recent study showed only two thirds

---

[107] Evans, W. St. Caron's Church, Tregaron. *Cambrian News.*
[108] Cohen, H. Letter. William Evans papers.
[109] Bennett, J. R. Chest pain: heart or gullet? *Brit.Med.Jr.* 1983. 286.1231.

The greatest pleasure of life is love

The greatest treasure

CONTENTMENT.

The greatest possession, health

The greatest ease is sleep

The greatest need is a TRUE FRIEND.

Sir William Temple.

of patients admitted to hospital because of anterior chest pain turned out to have ischaemic heart disease similar to the figure that William Evans had found in 1959. In a fifth of patients the pain may have originated in the oesophagus.

Harley Williams[110] has written that WE witnessed the historic operation on the mitral value by Sir Henry Souttar. This took place on Wednesday, 6 May 1925 when Souttar carried out the first trans-auricular mitral valvotomy for the relief of Mitral Stenosis, the anaesthetist being E. C. Lindsay. WE had been Dresser to Mr Souttar from 1 October to 31 December 1922.[111] He qualified with Honours in Surgery in June 1925 so although he wasn't on Mr Souttar's firm at the time he could well have been present as a witness. He was Assistant Anaesthetist to the Dental Department from 1 August to 27 November 1927 and had been Dresser to Mr E. C. Lindsay in 1922 so possibly was interested in anaesthesia at the time this surgery took place.

He didn't believe that cardiac surgery had a future and many of his opinions are dated and show him to have been wrong.

That does not detract from his papers many of which are outstanding but with the use of better apparatus and techniques knowledge increased.

Amongst the findings I uncovered when I was researching this book was that he had finished 'Back Home'. I was told that it was to be a sequel to his Autobiography but I later discovered that it had not been published. I discovered that it was Joseph Jenkins, his grandfather's biography mixed with the 'Trecefel Diaries' and not WE's autobiography.

My search to find a copy has so far been fruitless. After it had been turned down by his London publisher he took it to another but they also decided not to publish. Before WE had collected it from them a book appeared titled 'O Dregaron i Bangaroo' giving what I presumed to be a version of 'Back Home' in Welsh. When WE heard of this he went immediately to the publisher and threatened legal action unless the book was immediately withdrawn and shredded.

This was done but not before a few copies had been sold which have not been retrieved and so there are some copies available. The notes WE made for 'Back Home' are also not available for inspection.

---

[110] Williams, H. 'William Evans – Beloved Physician'. Health 1970. Summer. p. 31.
[111] Evans, William – Archives. Royal London Hospital.

This tantalising ending is the sort of puzzle which raises numerous questions and merits further investigation which Willie would have enjoyed for he would have revelled in finding out the truth.

Scope for a further story?

Another intriguing question is why did he not receive an Honour? Sceptics are surprised at the reason given, that he had pronounced Baldwin's heart healthy. Did he refuse to accept an Honour? I doubt it as there is no evidence. The reason may be altogether more complex. He was an Idealist, a man of high moral standing who commanded respect and a compassionate man who worked in the east End of London and saw at first hand Poverty and its effect on the population. I was told he never did anything wrong but did he in the 30's and 40's become involved in something to try and improve their lot which did not meet with Palace approval? I find that hard to believe for he had been appointed High Sheriff, had attended a Garden party in Buckingham Palace on 19 July 1955 and had met the Prince of Wales.

Whatever the reason it does not detract from his many achievements for he was one of Cardiganshire's most illustrious sons.

# APPENDIX I

## PRIZES GAINED AT LONDON HOSPITAL

1921   Surgical Dressers Prize (Hon.Cert.)
1922   Prize in Elementary Clinical Surgery
1927   K. E. D. Payne Prize in Pathology
1929   Hutchinson Triennial Prize in Clinical Surgery
1930   Liddle Triennial Prize in Pathology

# APPENDIX II

**Born:**

24.11.1895 – Tyndomen, Tregaron.

**Qualification:**

M.R.C.S., L.R.C.P. – Oct. 1924
M.B., B.S. – May 1925 (Hons.Surgery)
M.D. – 1927
M.R.C.P. – 1928
F.R.C.P. – 1935
D.Sc.(Lond.) – 1946
Hon.D.Sc.(Wales) – 1961

**Appointment:**

Consulting Physician London Hospital
The National Heart Hospital
Institute of Cardiology
(on staff of London Hospital 1926-1960)

1967 – Return to Tregaron

**Died:**

Withybush Hospital, Haverfordwest – 20.9.1988

Cremation – Marylebone.

Memorial Service Tregaron – 22.10.88

## APPENDIX III

**Meeting London Hospital Medical Council. 20 June 1934.**
Item: 4. At 9 o'clock consideration of applications and Testimonials
for Assistant Director of Medical Unit.

The Following was the result of the Ballot:–

|                  |    |
|------------------|----|
| Dr W. Evans      | 17 |
| Dr Aitken        | 10 |
| Dr Levy Simpson  | 4  |
| Dr Hoyle         | 2  |

**Meeting July 18th, 1934**
Item 2C. Dr William Evans was appointed Assistant Physician and
Assistant Director Medical Unit subject to confirmation by Court of
Governors.

*Signed:* Arthur G. Elliott, House Governor.

# APPENDIX IV

MEDICAL BOOKS
*Student Handbook of Clinical Electrocardiography* 1934
*Cardiology* 1948; 2nd Edition, 1956
*Cardioscopy* 1952
*Cardiography* 2nd Edition, 1954
*Diseases of Heart & Great Vessels* 1964

GENERAL BOOKS
*A Journey to Harley Street* 1969
*A Welsh Swagman* 1975
*Back Home* (not published)
*St. Caron's Church, Tregaron; Cambrian News.* No date.
*Need I Ever Retire?* – Chest and Heart Association 1965
*100 Scientific Papers* (41 in *British Heart Journal*)

# APPENDIX V

MEMORIAL LECTURES

Strickland Goodall Lecture – Society of Apothecaries, London 1942.

Finalyson Lecture – Glasgow, 1947.

St. Cyres Lecture – National Heart Hospital, London, 1952.

Gerrish Milliken Lecture – Philadelphia, 1954.

First Rufus Stolp Lecture – Evanston, Illinois, 1954.

Carbutt Lecture – Guy's Hospital, London, 1957.

Wiltshire Lecture – King's College Hospital, London, 1961.
'To tell Trash from Treasure'

Schorstein Memorial Lecture – London Hospital, 1961.
'Cardiology at the London Hospital'

First Leonard Abrahamson Lecture – Royal College of Surgeons, Dublin, 1963. 'Whither Cardiology?'

The Sir Thomas & Lady Dixon Lecture – '40 years in Cardiology', 1965.

# APPENDIX VI

## HONORARY MEMBER
British Cardiac Society in 1961.
Australian & New Zealand Cardiac Society.
American Cardiac Society.
Society of Physicians of Wales.
Honorary Fellowship of the Royal Society of Medicine 1976
(these are given to those who have distinguished themselves
in the Service of Medicine and branches of Science allied to
it)

## HONORARY CONSULTING CARDIOLOGIST
Messrs. Lloyds Bank
Royal Navy.
Royal Society of Musicians.
General Post Office

## HONOURED IN WALES
High Sheriff of Cardiganshire, 1959-60.
Hon. Members of the Order of Druids of the Royal National
Eisteddfod – Amnon III, 1960.
Honorary D.Sc. – University of Wales, 1961.
Member Court of Governors UCW Aberystwyth.

## HONOURS
1948 – Founder President British Soc. of Cardiological
Technicians .
1954 – First recipient Sydney Gold Medal for work in
Cardiology.
1980 – Elected 'Knight of Mark Twain' in recognition of his
outstanding contribution to modern medical science.
1976 – Hon. Fellow – R.S.M.

## FOUNDER MEMBER
British Cardiac Society, 1937. Member Council 42-46, 56-60,
Chair. 1965.
British Society of Cardiological Technicians, 1948.

# APPENDIX VII

## B.H.F.

Dinner at Lord Horace Evans' home
17th July, 1961

**Present:**
Lord Evans, Chairman
Dr Harley Williams
Sir John Mellor
Sir Eric Mieville
Mr Harold Samuel
Mr Lazell
Mr Forte
Mr Colin Coote
Mr Harold Peake
Lord Drogheda
Sir Ivan Stedeford
Mr Harry Moore
Lord Knollys
Lord Rank
Mr Simon Combe
Lord Cobbold
Mr Edward Thompson
Hon. Gavin Astor
Dr William Evans

# APPENDIX VIII

OBITUARIES

| | |
|---|---|
| Evans, B. | William Evans, *British Heart Journal*. 1989. 61: 68-70. |
| David, T. | 'Hearts but no Coronets' Plane 72 Dec/Jan. 88/89. |
| Mendel, D. | William Evans, *Independent Newspaper* 24.9.1988. |
| Newyddion | 'Un o Gewri'r Galon' *Golwg* 1988. Cyfrol 1; Rhif 5; Tud. 6 |
| Obituary | William Evans, *Times* 22.9.88. |
| Obituary | William Evans, *The Daily Telegraph* 27.9.88. p. 25. |
| Obituary | William Evans, *Cambrian News* 30.9.88. |
| Obituary | Death of renowned heart specialist, *Western Mail* 22.9.88. |
| Rhys,W.J.StE–G. | William Evans. *The Lancet* 10.12.88. p. 1376. |
| Towers, M. | William Evans, 'A true student of the tell-tale heart' *Guardian* 28.9.88. |
| Towers, M. | William Evans, *The Lancet* 8.10.88, p. 859. |

# APPENDIX IX

1. SEVERE ANAEMIA OF PREGNANCY AND THE PUERPERIUM. *Lancet,* 1929, **1,** 14.
2. POST-OPERATIVE GASTRIC ACIDITY. (with E. C. Lindsay). *Lancet,* 1929, **1,** 651.
3. BANTI'S SYNDROME AND 'SPLENIC ANAEMIA. *London Hospital Gazette,* June 1929.
4. GAUCHER'S DISEASE THIRTEEN YEARS AFTER SPLENECTOMY. (with D. Hunter). Proc. Roy. Soc. Med., 1929, **23,** 24.
5. INTRASACRAL EPIDURAL INJECTION IN THE TREATMENT OF SCIATICA. *Lancet,* 1930, 2, 1225.
6. THE PATHOLOGY AND ETIOLOGY OF BRAIN ABSCESS. *Lancet,* 1931, **1,** 1231 and 1289.
7. PARADOXICAL EMBOLISM. (with T. Thompson). *Quart. J. Med.,* 1930, **23,** 135.
8. A BRIEF HISTORY OF THE CARDIAC DEPARTMENT OF THE LONDON HOSPITAL. *London Hospital Gazette,* October 1931.
9. CONGENITAL STENOSIS (COARCTATION), ATRESIA, AND INTERRUPTION OF THE AORTIC ARCH. (A Study of 28 cases). *Quart. J. Med.,* 1933, **2,** 1.
10. THE EFFECTS OF NITRITE ON THE INVERTED T WAVE IN THE HUMAN ELECTROCARDIOGRAM. (with C. Hoyle). *Lancet,* 1933, **1,** 1109.
11. HARMOL HYDROCHLORIDE AND O-N-PROPYLHARMOL LACTATE IN ANGINA PECTORIS. (with C. Bramwell and M. Campbell). *Lancet,* 1933, **2,** 69.
12. THE COMPARATIVE VALUE OF DRUGS USED IN THE CONTINUOUS TREATMENT OF ANGINA PECTORIS. (with C. Hoyle). *Quart. J. Med.,* 1933, **26,** 311.
13. THE PREVENTION AND TREATMENT OF INDIVIDUAL ATTACKS OF ANGINA PECTORIS (ANGINA OF EFFORT). (with C. Hoyle). *Quart. J. Med.,* 1934, **27,** 105.
14. THERAPEUTIC EFFECT OF A PERIOD OF REST IN BED IN ANGINA PECTORIS (ANGINA OF EFFORT). (with C. Hoyle). *Lancet,* 1934, **1,** 563.
15. THE COURSE OF THE OESOPHAGUS IN HEALTH, AND IN DISEASE OF THE HEART AND GREAT VESSELS. *Med. Res. Coun, Spec. Rep. Series,* 1936, No. 208.
16. CARDIOVASCULAR DISORDERS. *Practitioner,* 1936, **137,** 441.

17. EARLY DIAGNOSIS AND TREATMENT OF HEART FAILURE. *Brit. Med. J.,* 1937, **1,** 1145.
18. THE NEWER ELECTROCARDIOGRAM DENOTING RIGHT BUNDLE-BRANCH BLOCK. (with H. M. Turnbull). *Lancet,* 1937, **2,** 1127 and 1184.
19. VITAMIN C IN HEART FAILURE. *Lancet,* 1938, **1,** 308.
20. CARDIOVASCULAR DISEASES. *Brit. Encyc. Med. Pract.,* 1939, 56.
21. THE DRUG TREATMENT OF HYPERPIESIA. (with O. Loughnan). *Brit. Heart. J.,* 1939, **1,** 199.
22. THE RELATIVE VALUE OF CERTAIN DIGITALIS PREPARATIONS IN HEART FAILURE WITH AURICULAR FIBRILLATION. *Brit. Heart J.,* 1940, **2,** 51.
23. A COMPARISON OF THE MERCURIAL DIURETICS USED IN HEART FAILURE. (with T. Paxton). *Brit. Heart J.,* 1941, **3,** 112.
24. THE ELECTROCARDIOGRAM OF STOKES-ADAMS ATTACK. (with J. Parkinson and C. Papp). *Brit. Heart J.,* 1941, **3,** 171.
25. CHEST LEAD ELECTROCARDIOGRAMS IN AURICULAR FIBRILLATION. *Brit. Heart J.,* 1941, **2,** 247.
26. CARDIOVASCULAR DISEASES. *Brit. Encyc. Med. Pract.,* 1942, 44.
27. THE ELECTROCARDIOGRAM IN FRIEDREICH DISEASE. (with G. Wright). *Brit. Heart J.,* 1942, **4,** 91.
28. MITRAL SYSTOLIC MURMURS. *Brit. Med. J.,* 1943, **1,** 8.
29. EMBOLISM. *Practitioner.* 1943, **150,** 148.
30. CHEST LEAD $CR_7$ IN CARDIAC INFARCTION. (with A. Hunter). *Brit. Heart J.,* 1943, **5,** 73.
31. TRIPLE HEART RHYTHM. *Brit. Heart J.,* 1943, **5,** 205.
32. THE HEART IN MYOTONIA ATROPHICA. *Brit. Heart J.,* 1944, **6,** 41.
33. THE UNITY OF PAROXYSMAL TACHYCARDIA AND AURICULAR FLUTTER. *Brit. Heart J.,* 1944, **6,** 221.
34. THE CAROTID SHUDDER. (with D. Lewes). *Brit. Heart J.,* 1945, **7,** 171.
35. THE HEART IN STERNAL DEPRESSION. *Brit. Heart J.,* 1946, **8,** 162.
36. PRIMARY PULMONARY HYPERTENSION. (with J. R. Gilmour). *J. Path. Bact.,* 1946, **58,** 687.
37. HEART MURMURS. *Brit. Heart J.,* 1947, **9,** 1 and 225.
38. CARDIAC PAIN. *Med. Soc. Lond. Trans.,* 1947, **65,** 295.
39. CARDIAC PAIN. Address at the Royal Melbourne Hospital, 1948.
40. MASS THROMBUS OF THE LEFT AURICLE. (with R. Benson). *Brit. Heart J.,* 1948, **10,** 39.

41. RAPID DIGITALISATION. (with P. Dick and B. Evans). *Brit. Heart J.,* 1948, **10,** 103.
42. THE SIMULATION OF HEART DISEASE. Proc. Roy. Australasian Col. Phys., 1948, **3,** 101.
43. FAMILIAL CARDIOMEGALY. *Brit. Heart J.,* 1949, **11,** 68.
44. THE HEART IN ENDOCRINE DISEASE. *Proc. Roy. Soc. Med.,* 1949, **42,** 331.
45. TRIPLE HEART RHYTHM AS A SIGN OF CARDIAC PAIN. *Lancet,* 1949, **2,** 737.
46. INNOCENT MURMURS. *Brit. Encyc. Med. Pract.,* 1949, **6,** 275.
47. THE USE AND ABUSE OF THE ELECTROCARDIOGRAPH. *Practitioner,* 1949, 162, 110.
48. HEART DISEASE IN CHILDREN. Public Health, October 1949.
49. THE USE OF THE PHONOCARDIOGRAPH IN CLINICAL MEDICINE. *Lancet,* 1951, **1,** 1083.
50. CONGENITAL PULMONARY HYPERTENSION. *Proc Roy. Soc. Med.,* 1951, **44,** 600.
51. THE EFFECT OF DEEP INBREATHING ON LEAD III OF THE ELECTROCARDIOGRAM. *Brit. Heart. J.,* 1951, **13,** 457.
52. CONSTRICTIVE PERICARDITIS. (with F. Jackson). *Brit. Heart J.,* 1952, **14,** 53.
53. THE LESSER ELECTROCARDIOGRAPHIC SIGNS OF CARDIAC PAIN. (with C. McRae). *Brit. Heart J.,* 1952, **14,** 429.
54. OESOPHAGEAL CONTRACTION AND CARDIAC PAIN. *Lancet,* 1952, **2,** 1092.
55. LONE AURICULAR FIBRILLATION. (with P. Swann). *Brit. Heart J.,* 1954, **16,** 189.
56. ANTICOAGULANT THERAPY IN CORONARY ARTERY OCCLUSION. *Proc. Roy. Soc. Med.,* 1954, **47,** 318.
57. THE DISTINCTIVE ELECTROCARDIOGRAM OF CORONARY ARTERIOSPASM. *Brit. Heart J.,* 1955, **17,** 15.
58. PAINLESS CARDIAC INFARCTION. (with G. C. Sutton). *Brit. Heart J.,* 1956, **18,** 259.
59. SOLITARY PULMONARY HYPERTENSION. (with D. S. Short and D. E. Bedford). *Brit. Heart J.,* 1957, **19,** 93.
60. THE SYNDROME OF THE SUSPENDED HEART. (with H. G. Lloyd-Thomas). *Brit. Heart J.,* 1957, **19,** 153.
61. CONDITIONS THAT MIMIC HEART DISEASE. *Guy's Hospital Gazette,* July 1957.

62. HYPERTONIA OR UNEVENTFUL HIGH BLOOD PRESSURE. *Lancet,* 1957, **2,** 53.

63. ADDITIONAL ELECTROCARDIOGRAPHIC SIGNS OF CARDIAC PAIN. (with R. K. Pillay). *Brit. Heart J.,* 1957, **19,** 366.

64. PULMONARY HYPERTENSION IN MITRAL STENOSIS. (with D. S. Short). *Brit. Heart J.,* 1957, **19,** 457.

65. PULMONARY HYPERTENSION IN CONGENITAL HEART DISEASE. (with D. S. Short). *Brit. Heart J.,* 1958, **20,** 529.

66. POLYTHELIA IN CARDIO-ARTERIAL DISEASE. *Brit. Heart J.,* 1959, **21,** 130.

67. FAULTS IN THE DIAGNOSIS AND MANAGEMENT OF CARDIAC PAIN. *Brit. Med. J.,* 1959, **1,** 249.

68. THE LESS COMMON FORMS OF PULMONARY HYPERTENSION. *Brit. Heart J.,* 1959, 21, 197.

69. THE DIAGNOSIS AND TREATMENT OF CARDIAC INFARCTION. J. Irish Med. Assoc., 1959, **45,** 34.

70. ON GIVING AND TAKING MEDICINES. *London Hospital Gazette,* May 1959.

71. THE ELECTRCARDIOGRAM OF ALCOHOLIC CARDIOMYOPATHY. *Brit. Heart J.,* 1959, 21, 445.

72. THE ETIOLOGY OF SYSTEMIC HYPERTENSION. *Brit. Heart J.,* 1960, **22,** 17.

73. MYOCARDIAL INJURY FROM THERAPEUTIC IRRADIATION. (with M. Catterrall). *Brit. Heart J.,* 1960, **22,** 168.

74. THE SIGNIFICANCE OF DEEP S WAVES IN LEADS II AND III. (with H. Davies). *Brit. Heart J.,* 1960, **22,** 551.

75. THE MANAGEMENT OF PAROXYSMAL ATRIAL FIBRILLATION. *Prog. Cardiovasc. Dis.,* 1960, **2,** 480.

76. DIGITALIS THERAPY. *Practitioner,* 1961, **186,** 3.

77. THE VOWS YOU HAVE BROKEN. *London Hospital Gazette,* March 1961.

78. ALCOHOLIC CARDIOMYOPATHY. *Amer. Heart J.,* 1961, **61,** 556.

79. THE INFREQUENT NORMAL ELECTROCARDIOGRAM IN CARDIAC PAIN. (with H. G. Lloyd-Thomas). *Amer. Heart J.,* 1961, **62,** 51.

80. CARDIOLOGY AT THE LONDON HOSPITAL. *London Hospital Gazette,* October 1961.

81. ELECTROCARDIOGRAPHY AS A MEANS OF PRESAGING CARDIAC PAIN. *Brit. Heart J.,* 1961, **23,** 669.

82. TO TELL TRASH FROM TREASURE. *King's College Hospital Gazette,* December 1961.

83. THE ELECTROCARDIOGRAM IN THE DIAGNOSIS OF SYSTEMIC HYPERTENSION. *Brit. Heart J.*, 1962, **24,** 469.

84. WHICH LEADS SHALL WE TAKE? *Amer. Heart J.*, 1962, **64,** 143.

85. ADDICTION TO MEDICINES. *Brit. Med. J.*, 1962, **2,** 722.

86. DIFFUSE ARTERIOPATHY. BRIT. HEART J., 1962, **24,** 703.

87. PITFALLS IN CARDIAC DIAGNOSIS. *Practitioner,* 1963, **190,** 177.

88. HYPERTENSION: MANAGEMENT AND RESULTS. *Proc. Roy. Soc. Med.,* 1963, **56,** 405.

89. CARDIOGRAPHIC CONTRECOUP IN THE COURSE OF CARDIAC INFARCTION. *Brit. Heart J.*, 1963, **25,** 725.

90. WHITHER CARDIOLOGY? *J. Roy. Coll. Surg.* Ireland. 1963, **1,** 13.

91. THE CURRENT STATE OF DIGITALIS. *Practitioner.* 1964, **193,** 368.

92. ALCOHOLIC MYOCARDIOPATHY. *Prog. Cardiovasc. Dis.,* 1964, **7,** 151.

93. ABOUT RETIREMENT. Geront. *Clinica,* 1964, **6,** 278.

94. THE RIGHT OBLIQUE TRANSTHORACIC ELECTROCARDIOGRAM. *Brit. Heart J.*, 1965, **27,** 252.

95. PRESAGING CARDIAC PAIN. *Brit. Heart J.*, 1965, **27,** 856.

96. PAVING THE LAST MILE. Geront. *Clinica,* 1965, **7,** 247.

97. EMPLOYMENT AND REHABILITATION OF PATIENTS WITH HEART DISEASE. B.C.R.D. International Seminar, Oxford 1965.

98. ALCOHOL AND THE HEART. *Practitioner.* 1966, **196,** 238.

99. FORTY YEARS IN CARDIOLOGY. *Ulster Med. J.*, 1965, **35,** 111.

100. SIGNIFICANCE OF S WAVES IN LIMB LEADS II AND III OF THE ELECTROCARDIOGRAM. *Brit. Heart J.*, 1966, **28,** 829.

# APPENDIX X

## QUOTATIONS FROM THE LIPS OR PEN OF
## WILLIAM EVANS

*General:*

No patient should be the worse for seeing a doctor.

Every doctor should ensure that onetime he becomes a patient. Not till then is his medical education complete.

It is not bad manners to speak of good manners, especially bedside manners.

Should a garrulous patient frustrate your examination of him, take his mouth-temperature.

The clinician seeks the truth in his patient; the pathologist (i.e. morbid anatomist) has the stark truth before him.

Babinski never drank morning coffee. (Encouraging students to spend their time examining patients in the wards, where they may chance on a new clinical sign.

There is no loss so finite as lost opportunity; the search for it is futile.

To search and not to find is to find other things.

Perserverence is passport to success.

Science is to learn what Nature reveals. Research is to seek the secrets which she may be loathe to reveal.

When a new truth is unpalatable, it is paraded as unorthodox.

Example is mother's milk for the child, and essential nutrient for the medical student.

Human Nature is a convenient repository into which we may cast any of our accountable sins.

One's past is either the dust-bin of lost opportunities, or the granary of accumulated wisdom.

The industrious fill the hour and would feign extend it.

Leisure is opportunity to do work which we have left undone.

Leisure is ill-spent unless it gathers treasure other than pleasure.

Immortality depends largely on other people's memories.

Silence is the mind's playtime.

To understand is to heed the opposite.

Many thoughts are silent for too long; others were best unspoken.

When sentiment is in the van, the heart governs the mind.

A hunch often steers the research-worker to the truth.

No-one should write a book unless he has a message to convey; too many books are message-less.

Books, the written thoughts of men, are placed to hibernate on shelves, for charwomen to dust.

Advice is seldom taken unless consonant with one's own opinion.

Euthanasia is murder glossed-over.

Research in medicine should be directed either to Diagnosis or Treatment; all else is twaddle.

The sage reasons; fools argue.

All is controlled. Birth is controlled, finance managed, production regulated. All is disciplined except self. Self-control is taboo.

Better health than wealth. (Motto on WE's crest as High Sheriff)

Perfection is for pursuit rather than capture, for aspiration not possession.

The child likes school the least; when grown to adult, regrets it most.

Defeat is but a stimulus to do better. Failure is often the first step to success.

Physical work is welcomed rest for the mind.

Memory is best companion in loneliness.

To correct one's own error is insurance against committing another.

To the question why she liked making beds, the nurse replied, 'They look so nice when they are finished.' – A fitting motto for all work.

A chance happening gains glory when its true meaning surfaces. (Witness the discovery of penicillin as an example of serendipity)

Time was before creation.

Tears do not come from the eyes, but from the heart, albeit a broken heart.

Shun smoking because it is an unsavoury habit, and not because it ever causes heart disease through encouraging the growth of coronary atheroma.

*Statistics:* That artful art which gives a scientific slant to changing possibilities to probabilities, converting fancies into facts, shadows into substance, and beliefs needing a pinch of salt into one having less than a grain of truth: I say, get thee behind me Satan!

Latin is going out of Oxford, and there is grave danger that good doctoring is going out of Medicine.

Criticism is a prerogative of leadership, not of discipleship.

Age buys experience, and experience in medicine is a precious commodity.

'We have always done it this way', is a cry against change, and often it has proved sounder doctrine than a call for so-called progress.

It is they, where illness has bared the fangs of death, that most appreciate recaptured health.

The fear of death is greater torment than dying.

Death is like sleep, but longer.

Death is the cure for an incurable illness.

To be health-conscious is to be out of health.

Concern for health places health at risk.

To face facts is to forsake cant.


## Diagnosis:

Do not view the Electrocardiogram through sightless eyes; small changes can presage grave events.

'Percussion has added nothing to cardiology in the last century,' so said John Parkinson, and I would add, nor will it during the next.

Intuition may prove a useful beacon in diagnosis, but don't let it dazzle you.

Never act on first impressions, but don't discard them; keep them aside but safe; they often prove to be the true diagnosis.

The diagnosis of a 'Tired heart', exposes the tired mind of the diagnostician.

Gaze long at the venous pulse in the neck, that natural manometer which records the movements and pressures in the right heart.

Keep close to the patient, at the head and not at the foot of the bed. The
Good Physician of Gallilee laid hands on those whom He
healed.

When the patient is being examined, there are two people at work;
while the doctor is searching for a diagnosis, the patient is
summing up the doctor. (In the case of the Psychiatrist, the
patient usually gets there first).

The art of auscultation depends on listening more than hearing.

It is an advantage to a cardiologist to be a little deaf. (Speaking of the
innocent systolic murmur).

When a student auscultates the heart, his lips should be moving as
evidence that he is truly at work, engaging in self-catechism.

The two phases of systole and diastole should be auscultated
separately, consecutively, and never concurrently.

To diagnose a systolic murmur in the mitral area as Mitral
Incompetence is incompetence but not mitral.

When two or more clinicians demur on the diagnosis of a cardiac
condition, consider Bacterial Endocarditis.

A multiplicity of electrocardiographic leads, leads to duplicity in
interpretation.

The attraction of ingenious machines, and fascination of complicated
laboratory tests, have captivated the faith and trust of the unwary
doctor, to make him less wary of his true function as a bedside
physician, a clinician.

There are signs that we are getting our fun out of medicine. Man is
being preferred to the rat for investigation, and for two reasons,
he is a more docile animal and has better veins.

To arrive at a diagnosis through complex rather than simple means , is
a pervading sin of present-day medicine.

The sphygmomanometer confounds more often than it aids diagnosis, not that it records incorrectly, but that the values it registers are so often misinterpreted.

### *Treatment:*

'Tis better to do nothing than something when nothing needs to be done.

Planned hesitancy before a deed to be done, is insurance that it needs to be done, and that it is well done. Precipitancy in treatment is usually bad therapy.

Healing is a slow ritual; it needs time.

Physical work is best for resting the mind.

In retirement from work, if anything stays, let work stay.

Loneliness as a lone illness is a preventable disease; its specific antidote is continued occupation.

Never decry digitalis.

Lean meat is for the limp and languid, the fickle, the faddy and the fanciful, who fear fatty foods, and favour the fast for the feast.

Model advice on diet; arise from the table feeling you could eat more.

Medical students should grow to be lean doctors so that they may chide their obese patients.

Concerning the oral use of long-acting nitrites, the only long-acting thing here, is the gullibility of those who prescribe them.

The relentless therapist should be aware of the moment when man has a right to die.

To practise proper medicine requires time; a hurried or tired physician is ill-equipped to infuse hope and courage into a dejected patient.

In the treatment of heart disease it is well to remember that the mind and heart are close companions, and attention to the former, is often the first need.

Just as superstition thwarts religion, so does quackery bedevil medicine. Every diktat of the former, and coloured pill of the latter, are swallowed as hallowed preservers of the soul in one case and the body in the other.

To work hard during each day, spares the discomfort of sleeplessness at night. The dignity belonging to work, and the health-giving property of work, need to be shouted from the house-tops.

We must talk more to our patients. So often, and more often, words are better therapeutic agents than medicines. To be dumb at a patient's bedside is to miss the opportunity to make him better.

The ruthless therapist in his obduracy and inordinate haste, fails to acquaint himself with the natural history of disease, and so remains ignorant of 'vis medicatrix naturae', the healing power of Nature.

Through the years, I have been amazed at the healing properties of coloured water, especially the red kind.

Among the many medicaments which doctors carry in their bags, there can be none more precious than the pill, *'Reassurance'*, precious in that it is the one he has to use most frequently.

Reassurance must always be unqualified reassurance, *'Reassurance without Strings'*. Not as happened in three of my patients who had successfully passed through an attack of coronary thrombosis. The doctor had said: –

*1st patient:* 'You have done well, but don't go out by yourself.'

*2nd patient:* 'You will be alright now, provided you don't get another one.'

*3rd patient:* 'Yes of course you may play golf, but don't walk uphill.'

Just as we have 20 digits on our hands and feet, we only need 20 drugs to do battle with any disease; these from the 2,000 listed in MIMS; the rest could be scrapped.

Retort to the H.P. who suggested anticoagulants to a patient with coronary thrombosis, 'I don't give rat poison to my patients.'

When anticoagulants went out of favour for this condition, – 'We rejoice in its outgoing; someone tried hard to prevent its incoming'.

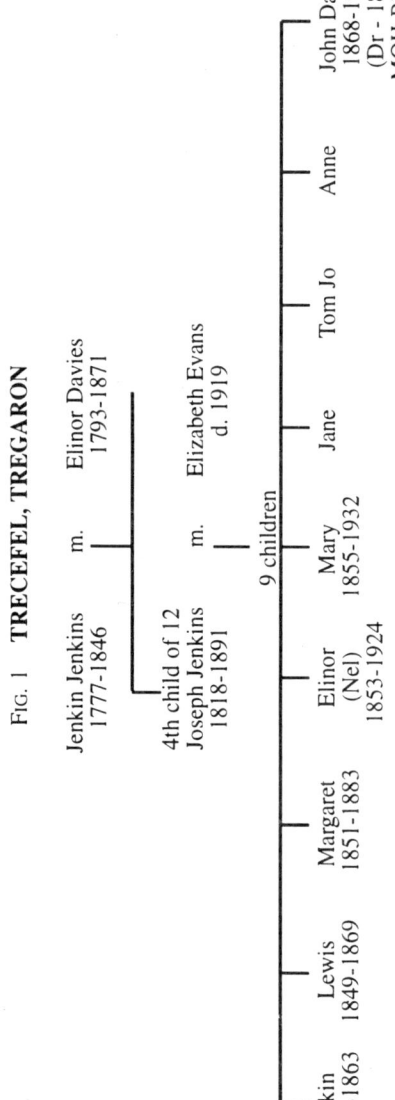

Fig. 1  **TRECEFEL, TREGARON**

Jenkin Jenkins       m.       Elinor Davies
1777-1846                      1793-1871

4th child of 12
Joseph Jenkins       m.       Elizabeth Evans
1818-1891                      d. 1919

9 children

Jenkin        Lewis        Margaret        Elinor        Mary        Jane        Tom Jo        Anne        John David
1846-1863     1849-1869    1851-1883       (Nel)         1855-1932                                        1868-1948
                                           1853-1924                                                      (Dr - 1893)
                                                                                                          MOH-Rhondda

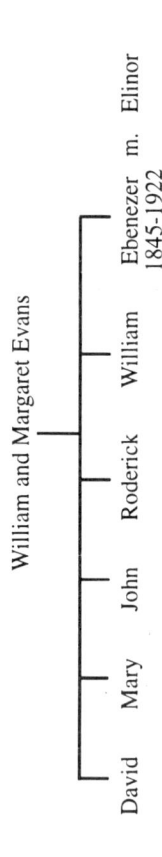

Fig. 2  **CRYNFRYNBYCHAN, LLANGEITHO**

William and Margaret Evans

David        Mary        John        Roderick        William        Ebenezer   m.   Elinor
                                                                     1845-1922

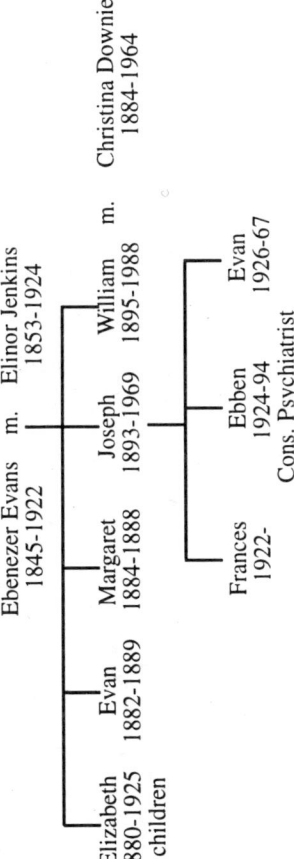

FIG. 3 **TYNDOMEN, TREGARON**